more than a body

more than a body

Your Body Is an Instrument, Not an Ornament

Lexie Kite, PhD, and Lindsay Kite, PhD

Houghton Mifflin Harcourt
Boston   New York
2020

For information about permission to reproduce selections from this book, write to trade.permissions@hmhco.com or to Permissions, Houghton Mifflin Harcourt Publishing Company, 3 Park Avenue, 19th Floor, New York, New York 10016.

hmhbooks.com

Library of Congress Cataloging-in-Publication Data
Names: Kite, Lexie, author. | Kite, Lindsay, author.
Title: More than a body : your body is an instrument, not an ornament / Lexie Kite, PhD, and Lindsay Kite, PhD
Description: Boston : Houghton Mifflin Harcourt, 2020. | Includes bibliographical references and index.
Identifiers: LCCN 2020034216 (print) | LCCN 2020034217 (ebook) | ISBN 9780358229247 (hardback) | ISBN 9780358393849 | ISBN 9780358393856 | ISBN 9780358226819 (ebook)
Subjects: LCSH: Body image. | Beauty, Personal—Psychological aspects. | Self-esteem in women. | Identity (Psychology)
Classification: LCC BF697.5.B63 K58 2021 (print) | LCC BF697.5.B63 (ebook) | DDC 306.4/613—dc23
LC record available at https://lccn.loc.gov/2020034216
LC ebook record available at https://lccn.loc.gov/2020034217

Book design by Chloe Foster

Printed in the United States of America
3 2021
4500833819

Contents

Introduction

No one experiences having their bodies and faces enthusiastically and unapologetically ogled, scanned, and compared by both strangers and loved ones like identical twins. We grew up without questioning this near-daily practice and learned to patiently wait and smile while people identified any supposed differences between us that would help them distinguish Lindsay from Lexie. Lindsay had the rounder face and straighter teeth. Lexie was a half inch taller and had a mole on her nose. Sometimes Lexie was thinner, sometimes Lindsay was, and this never went unnoticed (by ourselves or anyone else). A half pound and half inch difference between us at age nine was fodder for one of us to taunt the other with accusations of "Fat pig!" and other creative terms for being "fat and ugly." Our mom would point out that we were being ridiculous since we looked exactly the same, but we each insisted that couldn't be true and that our sister was, in fact, a fat pig.

In middle school, we competed to see who could lose the most weight, eat the fewest carbohydrates, and exercise the most hours. In Lexie's thirteen-year-old journal, she wrote, "Lindsay and I made a contest. We will try to get more hours of exercise than the other. I think I'm ahead of Lindsay by like 2 hours I hope. Next week I'll start on the dieting part. I hope I can stay on it. We're going to camp in like 26 days and I want to be skinny. We're gonna go swimming so I gotta look good in a swimsuit. Also, swim team is starting soon and I gotta be skinny and fit for that."

For as long as we can remember, we lived with a near-constant awareness and fixation on how we appeared. This was a result of others searching our bodies and faces for any detectable differences and commenting on them every single day, as well as the fact that we each were also visually scanning our own identical counterpart every day, watching how she looked from different angles and in different actions, effectively seeing our own appearances at all times. We didn't know this constant, critical awareness of the way we looked was noteworthy, let alone that it had a negative effect on our quality of life, self-esteem, relationships, and health. It took us until graduate school to find out that our constant mental body monitoring had hurt us and that it had a name, for twins and un-twinned people alike: self-objectification.

Self-objectification occurs when people learn to view their own bodies from an outside perspective, which is a natural result of living in an environment where bodies are objectified. We grow up seeing idealized and sexualized female bodies presented in media as parts for others' viewing pleasure, even in the most mundane or unexpected circumstances. In 1975, film theorist Laura Mulvey coined the term "the male gaze" to describe the phenomenon of women being represented in media through the perspective of a heterosexual man, in which they are sexualized and depicted as passive objects of male attention or desire. This is objectification. We then learn to monitor and understand our own bodies from the same outside perspective. This is self-objectification.

When we are self-objectifying, our identities are split in two: the one living her life and the one watching and judging her. We become our very own self-conscious identical twin, an onlooker to ourselves, monitoring how we look rather than how we are feeling or what we are doing. We live, and we imagine how we look as we live, adjusting and contorting ourselves accordingly. We watch from afar as our bodies become our primary means of identity and value. ***Our feelings about and perceptions of our bodies — our body image — become warped into our feelings about how we appear to ourselves and others.*** We learn that the most important thing about women is their bodies, and the most important thing about women's bodies is how they look.

In our objectifying culture, in which a high priority is placed on appearance and in which some bodies are praised and valued while others are degraded and marginalized, your body image — your feelings about your body — is informed by a lifetime of messages tying a woman's worth to her appearance. Those same messages define what it looks like to have an acceptable body — from the roots in your hair to the color of your toenails. Your body image becomes something you perceive from the outside, like your critical twin onlooker. She is the little voice in your head whispering, "Fat pig!" while you're getting dressed or sitting in a classroom or boardroom deciding whether to raise your hand or speak up. She is the nagging checklist reminding you to suck in, fix your makeup, adjust your clothes, pose the right way, play up your best-looking parts, and on and on and on. For many people, learning about self-objectification leads to a serious "aha!" moment as they put a name to this invisible and unquestioned —yet all-too-familiar—experience of body monitoring their days away.

Never is this split identity phenomenon more apparent than when we ask women and girls the simple question "How do you feel about your body?" So, let's start there.

If you were asked right at this moment how you feel about your body, what would you say? Don't twist your answer to fit a mold you think we (or anyone else) want it to fit, for better or worse. Just spill it. How do you feel about your body, and why do you think you feel that way?

Write out your feelings as thoroughly as you can in a journal or notebook or other safe spot. Do the same with the questions at the start of each chapter. You'll refer back to your responses later, and you'll be glad you were honest and candid with yourself.

In our doctoral research among eighteen- to thirty-five-year-old women and in the online body image course we have offered for several years to girls and women ages fourteen and up, we started with that same simple question: *How do you feel about your body?* What we've found over and over is that when you ask women about their body image—in other words, how they feel about their bodies—you'll get a bunch of answers to a totally different question. Most will describe how they think they look, highlighting what they or others perceive as their worst flaws: belly rolls, love handles, cellulite, loose skin, flat chests, embarrassing bits to hide or fix. It's as if rather than being asked how they *feel* about their bodies, they were asked, "What do you most fear someone will *see* when they look at you?" Overwhelmingly, their answers reflected embarrassment, fear, anxiety, and pain.

Other answers reflected appreciation for natural or hard-won thinness, clear skin, toned arms, or appealing curves. It's as if they were asked, "What do you love for people to see when they look at you?" Though those might sound like better answers at first, we worry about what the future holds for these women. Women who feel positively about their bodies because of how they look often fall even harder into negative body image and shame when they no longer live up to the ideal, whether because of aging, illness, pregnancy, or any other cause. When your main source of confidence and validation isn't producing the same results it used to, that loss stings.

The descriptions women give us of how they feel about their bodies, whether fearing or fawning, also reflect distance and detachment, as if the women are outside observers of their own bodies. It's that twin phenomenon, in which our critical, objectifying onlooker becomes the judge of how we should feel about the bodies we live inside of. While your body image is not something that can be viewed or perceived from the outside, too many of us can't imagine our feelings about our bodies from any other perspective. This reveals a deeper problem with women's body images and self-worth than most people recognize, and one that popular "You are beautiful!" body-image campaigns are not capable of solving: ***Women are privileging an external view of their bodies over their own internal, first-person perspec-***

tive. It's as if we, as women, exist outside of ourselves — as if our bodies can be understood only through someone else's eyes.

Women's self-objectifying responses to the question of how they feel about their bodies aren't mistakes or misunderstandings of how body image functions: it's brainwashing. We see women, including ourselves, as bodies *first* and people *second*. Boys, men, and people of all gender identities are not immune to the phenomenon of self-objectification, but it is particularly rampant among girls and women or those presenting themselves in a traditionally feminine way. We are all at a severe disadvantage when our self-perceptions and body images are so deeply tied to how we look (or how we *think* we look). Too many of us not only feel awful about our looks, since we can never achieve or maintain the aspirational beauty ideals presented to us, but also feel awful about our dynamic, adaptive, miraculous bodies overall because all we care about is how they *look*. This is truly the root of negative body image. To add insult to injury, we will likely feel awful about our*selves* as a whole because we've learned that our bodies define our worth. The problem of negative body image then extends to overall negative self-image, becoming a more comprehensive problem than beauty-focused solutions can tackle.

So how do we fix this? The most popular strategy for promoting positive body image relies on messaging such as "All bodies are beautiful" or "All bodies are bikini bodies" or "Our flaws make us beautiful." Those ideas might provide a temporary mood boost and are catchy marketing slogans, but ultimately they don't get to the root of the problem. Regardless of how the definition of beauty expands, it's still being reinforced as the most important thing about us. A more effective approach to healing our body image issues needs to reflect the understanding that focusing on the appearance of our bodies *is the problem*. We provide a new definition: ***Positive body image isn't believing your body looks good; it is knowing your body is good, regardless of how it looks.***

Each of us has grown up in and experienced every second of life inside our own incredible bodies, and yet we judge and define how we *feel* about our bodies by how we *think* they *look* to others? That thought would be laughable if it weren't so cryable. When we can understand and relate directly to our bodies by experiencing our physical selves from the inside, rather than maintaining a limited outside perspective, we can *see more* in our bodies and ourselves — more than a body to be looked at, judged, consumed, and discarded. Desiring validation for your looks isn't bad — it is completely normal, and that positive attention can be very affirming. Beauty can be fun and a creative expression. But experiencing and valuing yourself as a whole, embodied human means making sure you aren't prioritizing validation from others above your own well-being, health, and happiness, and not prioritizing an external perspective of who you are. No more trying to squeeze ourselves into the narrow molds of our cultural beauty ideals, and no more trying to stretch our cultural beauty ideals to fit all of us. No more struggling to convince ourselves we are all beautiful since beauty is the greatest source of value and confidence we can imagine. Let's imagine something better than beautiful for ourselves and everyone we love.

Achieving peace with our bodies through developing positive

body image is the final frontier for too many women—the last and most stubborn barrier to our own confidence, fulfillment, power, and self-actualization. We can be empowered and emboldened and confident and successful in every other area of our lives, and yet still struggle with deep-seated body shame and self-objectification to which we sacrifice incredible amounts of time, money, emotion, and energy. While we have little control over the way others view and value us and the objectifying, dehumanizing, and demeaning environment that surrounds us, we do have control over the ways we respond to the pressures and pains that result.

In a culture that values some bodies and faces more than others, we recognize that some people confront much more significant barriers to developing a positive body image and pushing back on their own objectification. This is particularly true around intersections of race, ethnicity, gender and sexuality, class, ability, and body size that affect how people experience the world and how the world perceives their bodies. White women in particular need to be aware of their privilege in not being subject to, and sometimes perpetuating, the racial discrimination heaped upon women of color and the added appearance-related burdens placed upon Black women in particular. Women without disabilities need to be aware of the significant barriers women with disabilities of all kinds face in navigating a world that places such a premium on bodies that it renders visible disabilities invisible in most media. We all need to be aware of the significant backlash faced by many people who don't fit neatly into the stereotypical male/female binary or otherwise break gender norms in how they appear. Women who face body image burdens but can fit into most public seating and have easy access to clothing in their size need to understand that while body shame doesn't discriminate, women in larger bodies are tangibly and openly discriminated against and oppressed every day. When body image activism and campaigns center the bodies of women barely (or not at all) considered "plus-size," remember that those women aren't the ones facing the greatest stigma, even if they have also struggled.

None of us is immune to the harms of objectification, but it is important to acknowledge our own advantages that help alleviate the harshest aspects of that pain in our lives. We—Lexie and Lindsay—are white, middle class, heterosexual, educated, able-bodied women, and we recognize that despite hating our bodies for many years and falling short of body ideals in our culture, we also enjoy privileges that have protected us from any significant discrimination. These facets of our lives certainly play a role in our experiences within our own bodies and color our perspectives as activists and researchers. Though we've worked to learn from and incorporate a wide variety of perspectives, we acknowledge our privileges in a world that values whiteness, heterosexuality, middle-class status, and able bodies.

You'll notice that throughout this book, we primarily use female pronouns and speak to and about girls and women. This is because, from the beginning of our studies, we have maintained a narrow focus on female body image. We acknowledge that boys and men and nonbinary people also struggle with body image concerns. It is not our intention to exclude anyone, but to be clear about our specific research focus and findings rather than trying to claim expertise we don't have. However, we believe the concepts and strategies we illuminate in this book can be helpful to anyone who has experienced objectification and self-objectification, regardless of gender identity, sexuality, race or ethnicity, socioeconomic status, ability, nationality, or any other variable of difference. There may be parts of our work that don't seem to apply to your life or experiences, and we recognize that. We don't claim to have all the answers, but we do hope to offer some help for anyone who can benefit from our efforts.

In the chapters to follow, we aim to destabilize the normalness of seeing and being seen as objects in order to provide a more empowering path toward positive body image—starting with our framework for understanding not only the problem but also the solution: body image resilience. Starting in chapter 2, sections titled "See More" expose the messages and forces that keep us at home in a culture of objectification. Those titled "Be More" give you the resources and skills to hone a more positive body image and a stronger sense of self—one that prioritizes your whole identity, not just what is visible.

1

Rising with Body Image Resilience

- Describe an experience that caused a major disruption or shift in how you feel about your body. Your experience could be big or small, but it had a meaningful impact on your relationship with your body and how you saw yourself.
- What did you do to cope and manage your feelings about your body in response to that experience, whether positive or negative?

Every increment of consciousness, every step forward is a *travesia*, a crossing. I am again an alien in new territory. But if I escape conscious awareness, escape "knowing," I won't be moving. "Knowing" is painful because after "it" happens I can't stay in the same place and be comfortable. I am no longer the same person I was before.

—Gloria Anzaldúa, *Borderlands/La Frontera*

You are more than a body, and you knew that once. It takes some serious work to remember, understand, and experience this truth that you are more—more than beautiful, more than parts in need of fixing, more than an object to be looked at and evaluated. Can you remember when you *knew* you were more? When you lived free of that nagging concern for how you appeared? When how you looked had no influence on whether or not you joined in a game with friends or talked to someone or ran down the sidewalk? You might have to think back to some of your earliest memories, but take a few moments to remember a specific experience from your childhood when you were free from self-consciousness about how you looked or how others perceived you. If you can't come up with a memory, can you envision a photo or video of yourself of when you know you weren't fixated on your looks? Where were you? What were you doing? How did you feel?

For another glimpse into your past, spend time observing a young child. Watch them move, play, and speak freely. Imagine what that freedom must feel like. Try to remember what it did feel like. As you consider those feelings, you might experience longing, homesickness, regret, envy, or sadness for what once was and what might have been. These feelings are an important step in your body image path, so don't push them aside or numb them away. Let these emotions call out to you, inviting you down a liberating path back home to yourself.

The Sea of Objectification

Throughout this book, we will explore the forces that changed your body image and that of your "inner child" — what warped it into something you perceive only externally, and what split your identity into being simultaneously the seer and the seen. We then explore how to tap back into that early sense of body and self before you ventured away to evaluate yourself from afar. We invite you to envision this journey back home to yourself through the metaphor of a "sea of objectification," which splashes at your feet when you are very young, submerges you as you get older, and eventually becomes the only home you can remember or imagine. We are likening the phenomenon of objectification to a body of water because it is deep and wide-spanning, immersive, inviting, and both enjoyable and dangerous. It represents all of the ways women's bodies in particular are prized above all other aspects of their humanity and all of the ways women are taught they should look and act in order to be accepted, respected, valued, or desired. We can adapt and survive in the sea of objectification, but it is a constant burden on our mental and physical energy to keep our heads above water.

As little children, we all live on the sandy shore we'll refer to as More Than a Body Beach. Imagine yourself there as a child. You love the beach and spend your days having fun, playing in the sand, and watching the waves, all the while unaware and unburdened by how you appear to others. You have no anxiety about wearing a swimsuit or a big T-shirt and hat while slathered with thick sunscreen, no concern about what your stomach looks like as you hunch over a sandcastle, whether you have tan lines, or are sweaty, hairy, too exposed or not exposed enough, and on and on. From the shore, you can see the sea extends past the horizon. It looks inviting; lots of people are splashing and paddling in the water, encouraging you to wade in.

We all entered these waters at different times and through different means, whether by dipping a toe through browsing a family member's magazine collection out of curiosity, getting pushed in by a catcaller's lewd words or classmates' taunts of "fatso" or "beanpole," or even being swallowed up by a tsunami wave through sexual abuse. How did you first wade into the sea of objectification? Was it hearing your mom or sister talk about her own body in disparaging ways, and realizing you must need to look at your own body the same way? Was it watching a TV show that featured ideally beautiful female characters who didn't look like you or anyone you knew in real life? Was it the shock of hearing a man on the street yelling something at you or watching someone's eyes scan your body? Was it noticing which girls in your class got the most attention?

When you experience being objectified by others or become aware of the unavoidable objectification of bodies in our media, culture, and personal interactions, you learn to view yourself that way, and your identity becomes divided: the whole, embodied human on the beach, and the self-objectifying, image-focused part of yourself trying to stay afloat in the water. You leave behind your embodied, whole, complete self on the shore as you wade, dive, or get pulled into the water. As your clothes, skin, and hair get drenched, you are pulled into a new way of navigating and understanding the world and your place in it. Once you're in the water, you quickly start to become acclimated to it. After a while, it doesn't shock you or take your breath away anymore. It might even start to feel more comfortable than the air and land outside. You drift farther and farther from More Than a Body

Beach. We all grow up and grow older in various depths of this water, more often than not surrounded by others we know and love who entered the water before and after we did. We all adapt to it. We forget about our carefree inner children, whose lives and hopes and imaginations weren't distracted or limited by envisioning how they looked, and learn to cope with the demands of our new environment.

In the waters of objectification, you may have managed to find your own comfort zone when it comes to body image—sort of like settling in on a life raft. It may be flimsy, but it mostly keeps you afloat. It is the "normal" state of your body image, and it might not be all that comfortable. Think of the ways so many people respond to the question "How do you feel about your body?" (Discussed on page 36.) Their answers reveal deep discomfort and detachment from their own experiences in their bodies, but no one seems to think this is abnormal. Scholars describe this phenomenon as "normative discontent," meaning it is perfectly normal for girls and women to feel bad about our bodies most of the time. It feels natural to be uncomfortable with our bodies or to be constantly self-monitoring. If we do see the discomfort in our self-objectification and shame, we write it off as just another part of womanhood.

Many of us bond over that shared, normal discomfort with our bodies—what we hate, what we're trying to fix, how guilty we feel for eating or not exercising, and recruiting others to join our new plans for surefire success. Most of us can't even imagine what it might feel like to *not* exist this way—to be at home in our bodies instead of monitoring them from the outside, not constantly restricting and dieting or planning our next beauty fix or spend-ing time on everyday beauty "responsibilities" like makeup and fashion. You might not even consider body shame and appear-ance fixation to be problems because they are so seemingly *jus-tified*—after all, if you could simply muster enough self-control to abstain from sugar or carbs, or stick to your workout regimen, or not sleep on your side and not talk with so much expression to avoid all those wrinkles, you wouldn't have to worry about looking and feeling so awful. You become convinced that if you could just get it together, your body image would stay confidently afloat without the constant anxiety and exhaustion of failing on your diet or restarting a cardio routine after an indulgent vaca-tion or investing the time and money into the ultimate anti-aging regimen.

The solutions to your body image woes are advertised as being readily available in beauty fixes and straightforward diet plans, but the problem is always *you*—your weakness and lack of will-power. So you have grown comfortable with being uncomfort-able. You hate your body instead of hating the expectation that your body fit a certain mold. You hate your weakness and lack of discipline instead of hating the profit-driven solutions that are designed to require a lifetime of purchases but still leave you short of perpetually out of reach ideals.

Our uncomfortable body image life rafts never stay in one spot for long. They are collectively being pushed and pulled by currents of beauty-enhancing trends and changing body ideals. We often don't even recognize the currents that are carrying us around since almost everyone we can see is going in the same direction, just bobbing along in search of comfort and safety. Look through the most popular accounts on Instagram, and you'll see how homogenous and cohesive beauty and body ideals are at any point in time. When the same ideas of attractiveness are shared so widely and at such an incredible scale, it is no surprise that they shape our own body goals and preferences (for our own bodies and others'), carrying us along without our awareness that we're even moving. Some of the currents are more like dangerous riptides that can drag us under unexpectedly or sweep us away from places of peace or contentment. These all too prevalent riptides in the waters of objectification represent prejudice and bias against people who don't fit the ideals (fatphobia, racism, sexism, ageism, and classism) and dehumanization of women and girls that contributes to widespread violence and abuse. These invisible undercurrents shape our culture and make this environment much less safe and enjoyable for some than others.

Not everyone lives in the waters of objectification or faces the harms and dangers of spending time there. Some people—especially some men—are privileged to rarely be defined by or primarily valued for their appearance. Their identities never split into the object to be admired and the subject doing the admiring. They aren't dehumanized and objectified in any significant ways by others with more power. Men who don't fit appearance ideals are much less likely to face the repercussions women do because our culture values men for more than their bodies or their sexual desirability. Their looks are just *one part* of their identity, and rarely the most important part. Men are indeed valued for having an attractive appearance, but they are also valued for multiple aspects of their humanity, like intelligence, humor, talents, and accomplishments, regardless of how they look. Advantages like wealth and power also minimize the potential negative effects of being objectified for men who don't fit appearance ideals. Many men don't even know they have advantages protecting them from being pulled into the depths of the waters of objectification, and they (and we) might assume that those struggling in the currents of beauty ideals just need to work a little harder to reach a better destination or stay afloat.

Waves of Body Image Disruption

Whether or not we are comfortable in our body image "comfort zones," every one of us will still face life experiences and societal pressures that push us out of our life rafts. These waves of body image disruption—things like facing unreal ideals in media, aging, pregnancy, injury, illness, bullying, criticism, self-comparison, abuse, and violence—will knock you over, throw you for a loop, and shake up your relationship with your own body. Sometimes you see them coming, and sometimes you don't, like when a loved one comments on your weight and questions your eating habits, or when you see a photo of yourself that makes you feel ashamed. They can hit when you catch a glimpse of yourself in the mirror or see an ad hawking "body contouring" or the new fountain of youth or some procedure you secretly believe will fix your biggest problems, physical or otherwise. They can hit when you compare your body to someone else's (or to your own body in the past) or someone close to you becomes ultra-focused on their weight-loss plan or undergoes cosmetic surgery.

A severe body image disruption that pushes you out of your body image comfort zone might be the onset of a chronic illness that changes your entire outlook on your body, leaving you unable to do the things you've done before and changing your appearance in the process. It could be a devastating breakup or betrayal by a partner. It could be a sexual assault that distances you from your own body, leaving you feeling like your body is a weapon that was used against you. It could be a pregnancy or miscarriage that changes your body in ways you weren't prepared for while changing your lifestyle and relationships in the process.

These waves are big and small and different for everyone, but what they have in common is that they cause you to feel self-doubt, shame, fear, or anxiety about your body, and they demand your attention and response. We all respond to our body image disruptions in one way or another, but we often don't even think about how we react and what better options might be. Since getting pushed out of your comfort-zone life raft is not generally a positive experience, it is likely that you respond in ways that help you cope in the short term but maybe don't really serve you in the long term. As you think back on specific experiences when you felt increased body shame and self-objectification, ask yourself, "How did I cope?" We have identified three paths people take in response to body image disruptions, and they'll likely sound familiar to you from different points in your life or a loved one's.

Sinking into Shame

The first and worst path people take leaves them sinking into shame. Many of us deal with disruptions to our relationships with our bodies by numbing ourselves from having to feel pain or embarrassment, and when the distraction or numbness wears off, we are left in deeper pain, worse off than before. We may feel intense shame, despair, or depression, making it hard to engage with everyday life; at the most extreme end, these emotions can manifest in harmful behaviors. An alarming number of girls and women harm themselves through attempted suicide, cutting, overexertion, disordered eating, and abuse of alcohol and illegal and prescription drugs. When faced with the overwhelming pain of sexual or physical abuse, bullying and gossip, and rampant body shame and self-loathing, many girls and women admit to inflicting physical harm on themselves to punish themselves or numb their internal pain and shame. Others seek a temporary high to help them feel something new in the moment, only to push their internal agony back as long as they can.

Cutting and other forms of self-harm skew heavily female. Up to 30 percent of teenage girls in some parts of the United States say they have intentionally injured themselves without aiming to commit suicide, researchers have found. In 2019, about one in four adolescent girls deliberately harmed herself, often by cutting or burning, compared to about one in ten boys. Add to this the fact that self-harm among ten- to fourteen-year-old girls in the US has nearly tripled since 2009, according to the Centers for Disease Control and Prevention, and it is clear that girls are entering womanhood with deep pain and shame they are unable to deal with on their own.

The sheer number of teenage girls who come talk to us after our speaking events and admit to using self-harm as a coping mechanism is astounding. We have spoken with hundreds of girls over the years—in person and through email and messages— who deal with the agony of abuse, assault, bullying, and body shame by hurting themselves. They often couple their self-harm with disordered eating, and are eager to share when they hear us acknowledge their secret shame aloud. Their stories are nothing short of devastating, but they are not unique, and they have to be heard to be understood and addressed.

After reluctantly attending an event we spoke at in Tennessee, a thirteen-year-old girl shared with us her example of sinking into shame, writing:

"I used to cut myself. Well, my last time doing that was yesterday. But I did it because I was bullied about my looks. I was told to kill myself nearly every day. I was told that nobody would ever like me because of how I looked."

This is a heartbreaking example of coping through self-harm after the body image disruption of constant bullying.

After one of our speaking events in Idaho, a teenage girl emailed us that night to say:

"I have problems with going through stages and large periods of time where I don't eat, and I'm constantly judging myself and that's really all I've ever done for as long as I can remember. I hate myself more than anything and I've been self-harming for almost a year — I already have thousands of cuts and dozens of burns. I'm not sure if it's weird that I don't cut for the rush. I really don't feel any different before, during, or afterwards. I cut because I feel like I deserve pain and I can't kill myself because I feel like I would be cheating myself out of the pain I deserve to feel."

After speaking at an eating disorder treatment center, we received this email from a girl in attendance:

"Two years ago, I was raped by my boyfriend. At the time I was 15 and he was 23. I never hated my body more than after that horrible day. I couldn't even look in the mirror for the first few weeks. When I found out I was pregnant later I immediately let him know. He told me I had to get an abortion or he would 'ruin my life.' That night I attempted suicide. Finding out I lost the baby was my all-time low. I was so disgusted with myself, so horrified, that I don't even think words will ever have the ability to express it. There is no way to explain that pain. The next few months were absolute hell. I hopped from abusive relationship to abusive relationship, oftentimes taking part in the abuse myself."

None of these girls are alone in their secret, dark, sinking pain and shame, but they usually feel like they are. When our culture consistently portrays female bodies as parts served up on a platter to be used, evaluated, ogled, and cast aside, we can't blame them for internalizing that darkness and coping in dark ways that sink them deeper into shame. When feeling beautiful and desirable remains the only solution we can imagine to the large-scale problem of body image concerns, of course we are left feeling worthless and deserving of pain. And when you don't know other ways to deal with the brutal realities of life in this dehumanizing environment, and you don't feel worthy or equipped to seek better options, allowing yourself to sink to the bottom might feel like a reasonable response and the only one you are capable of making.

Clinging to Your Comfort Zone

The second path people take in response to a body image disruption is to try to "fix" their bodies. These quick fixes — such as buying new makeup or clothes, going on a liquid cleanse for the weekend, or making plans for or going through with cosmetic procedures like face fillers, lip injections, liposuction, or fat freezing — might temper your anxiety for a moment but don't offer lasting solutions. They alter the surface in an attempt to fix the "flaw" while simply postponing the necessity of dealing with your deeper body image concern. Your efforts might not even have any immediate effect on your appearance, but they give you the temporary feeling of control over your anxiety by creating or following through on a plan to fix your "problem areas." Many of the people we know are treading water right alongside us or being temporarily wooed toward mirages of confidence and positive body image through surefire solutions of weight loss/booty lifting/longer lashes/hairlessness/cellulite minimization/anti-aging efforts. The only problem is, this promised confidence and body love might not ever materialize, or will be only a temporary respite until the next "flaw" and "fix" is identified. Positive body image is an inside job. **When we keep attempting to fix an internal, mental problem with outside, physical solutions, those quick fixes will never really solve our problems,** nor will they prepare us to respond effectively to future body image disruptions.

When the "fixing" doesn't do the trick or your flaws seem too overwhelming to even try to change them, you might simply sit it out. You hide by opting out of anything that would require being seen.

From Lindsay: I remember the very first time I chose to hide myself rather than swim. I may have been embarrassed about how I looked before, but I had never let it overpower my desire to go swimming because it had been such a regular part of my life. Lexie and I had spent most of our childhood swimming, beginning with classes when we were very young, and then joining our city's swim team at age six. (The smell of chlorine still gets my heart racing, and reminds me of the weekends we spent traveling to swim meets and the practices before and after school.) My everyday life of swimming changed all at once when I was fifteen, a sophomore in high school, and taking a swimming class for PE credits at school with members of the swim team and other students. I had always been proud to be a swimmer, and I had already spent one semester loving my swimming class.

That all changed when I saw who else had joined the new class —cute, intimidating, older boys. My confidence in my swimming abilities was completely decimated by my fear of those boys seeing me in a swimsuit, judging the size of my thighs and the whiteness of my legs, seeing my eyes ringed by goggle lines, the makeup washed off my zit-prone chin. I was frozen, and I spent the first day of class sitting on deck, pretending I had forgotten my swimsuit. I spent every other day as the first person in the water and the last one out so no one could see me. I hid. I kept hiding.

Over the next several years, one of the most consistently jolting waves of disruption we both faced again and again came through a seemingly innocuous experience: being invited to go swimming. Though we were never insulted or bullied by anyone, we unleashed internal insults and bullying on ourselves each time we faced the opportunity to go to a pool, beach, hot tub, or lake. Rather than tell anyone the real reason we would never join them for a day at the pool, we listed off rapid-fire excuses while mentally making plans to fix ourselves so we could "qualify" to go next time. Our mouths said, "I've got too much to do, but definitely invite me next time!" or "I'm not feeling good, but have so much fun without me!" while our brains said, "No more carbs for you, and get ready for some serious treadmill time since you'd be humiliated if anyone saw you in a swimsuit this way!"

The problem with this response is that even when we hid inside to protect ourselves from the embarrassment we believed would overwhelm us, and even when we fixed or improved our supposed flaws through weight loss or hair removal or tanning or finding cute swimwear, we never felt any better about our bodies or ourselves. And when "next time" rolled around, we still declined.

Rising with Resilience

Here's the thing about body image disruptions: you always get to choose how you respond to them. You can fall into the same patterns of clinging to your comfort-zone life raft, trying quick fixes to keep your body image afloat, or simply hiding from the world. You can sink into shame and engage in self-destructive behavior. Or, you can follow the better—but often scarier—path: you can rise with resilience.

One of the unexpected benefits of facing waves of body image disruption is that they can remind you that you are in the waters of objectification—an environment that started out as a shock to your system at some point but over time became so normal it is invisible. They disrupt your body image comfort zone in ways you would never choose for yourself, but through your response to them, you can learn things about yourself and your environment that you can't learn any other way. *Difficult experiences and feelings about your body caused by objectification can work for you instead of against you.* The waves and currents can work as opportunities to not only *see more* in yourself and your environment, but also *be more* by pushing back on your normalized discomfort and dehumanization and working to change the dangerous conditions that surround you. This push to rise from the depths of shame and kick against currents of body expectations and pressures goes beyond simply coping and adapting to unideal circumstances. It requires more, and it produces more.

You have the capacity to not only survive your body image disruptions, but also grow and thrive and build strength and compassion and purpose *through* them. By developing your body image resilience, you gain the ability to access both innate and learned skills and strategies to both alleviate some of the pain caused by your disruptions and react to those waves in ways that improve your relationship with your body rather than push you further away from your whole, embodied self. You can recognize and work to overcome the negative effects of the objectification you might have come to accept as normal. Instead of coping in all the ways you used to, you can dig deep to learn from your experiences, to see more in them and in yourself, and to grow stronger, more capable, and more resilient.

Through our doctoral research, we realized the framework of resilience in positive psychology is a powerful approach to improving body image. Resilience, as both a trait and a process, is defined by one of the pioneers of this field of research (and one of our graduate school mentors), Glenn Richardson, as the process of "being disrupted by change, opportunities, adversity, stressors or challenges and, after some disorder, accessing personal gifts and strengths to grow stronger through the disruption." The resiliency model developed by Richardson illustrates three possible responses to deal with disruptions: reintegration with loss (or what we call sinking into shame), reintegration back to the comfort zone (or clinging to your comfort zone by hiding and fixing), and resilient reintegration (rising with resilience). This model helps illustrate how disruptions can be painful and throw us out of our comfort zones, but they can also make room for change, even when we don't know we need it. We can respond to the pain and shame we experience in ways that allow us to have "enabling" disruptions. After all, staying in our totally uncomfortable "comfort zones" doesn't require anything of us. No progress. No growth. Just hiding and fixing.

Our unique approach integrates research on objectification, body image, and resilience in order to explain and stop the frustrating cycle of self-objectification, in which women get stuck being evaluated by their appearance and then become their own evaluators, with few practical solutions to interrupt or end that cycle. Our steps for developing body image resilience will help you see and understand that objectification is all around us, but it doesn't have to be our internalized way of being. It doesn't have to split you in half as the seer and the seen, never being fully whole and at home in your own body.

That doesn't mean you can make the objectification of women, including yourself, just go away—it won't. It is persuasive and profitable, and it maintains hierarchies and inequalities enjoyed by people in power and those with the privilege to escape the harms of objectification. As long as we're surrounded by the waters of objectification, waves of disruption and currents of changing ideals and rampant prejudices will never stop. It is the nature of our environment. No matter how resilient and empowered you are, the reality is that discrimination, bias, prejudice, and culturally ingrained expectations of people—especially women, and especially women of color—still exist. Weight and size discrimination remains a stubbornly accepted prejudice in too many circles, even progressive ones. As Roxane Gay put it so succinctly in her book *Hunger,* "As a woman, as a fat woman, I am not supposed to take up space. And yet, as a feminist, I am encouraged to believe I can take up space. I live in a contradictory space where I should try to take up space but not too much of it, and not in the wrong way, where the wrong way is any way where my body is concerned."

In July 2019, activist Adrienne Hill posted publicly on Facebook about the burden of systemic weight bias in our culture, writing:

"I have been fat all my life, and I have been involved in fat activism since I was 19. During that time, I have done A LOT of body image work. But none of that body image work erases the pain of living in a fatphobic world. And yes, fat is a social justice issue. For me, it has meant not going to the doctor for years on end, and not getting the medical care I need, because I'm scared of getting a doctor who doesn't listen to me, who attributes all of my health problems to my weight, and who bullies me. It goes beyond the realm of medical care, too. Fat people have a harder time getting jobs, holding on to jobs, getting promotions, and so

on, because we live in a culture that presumes that a fat body says something about a person's work ethic. I'm really tired of being told that my objective experience of the world is, at its core, a self-esteem problem. I'm tired of having to constantly defend the idea that the injustices I face on the daily actually, objectively, exist; and that they're not my fault because I refuse to start the same endless cycle of yo-yo dieting that my mother did."

When body ideals and sex appeal are factors in women's evaluation by their employers, clients, students, doctors, family members, romantic prospects, and every stranger who passes by on the street or on the internet, women suffer. The burden is unbearable. That is truly a harsh reality of the objectifying culture we live in. Our recommendations for how people can respond to these disruptions and difficulties do not hinge on top-down solutions from government or other overseeing agencies (though we would love if those things happened), because we have little faith that those avenues will be successful. Instead, our research-backed methods for personal body image transformation count on all of us experiencing the sea of objectification and its associated stressors and then using those degrading and painful experiences as motivators to tap into our own power to rise with resilience regardless of whether or not our environment changes to meet us there. Through our individual and then collective action, we can gradually create a better and safer environment not only for ourselves, but for everyone else who deserves to see and be seen as more than a body.

In our efforts to offer help and solace to people seeking to improve their body image and our cultural ideas and realities around bodies, we acknowledge the work of pioneers in fat activism, who have tirelessly chipped away at the invisibility and injustice faced by people in larger bodies in all aspects of society. We also recognize the more mainstream body positivity movement's contributions to helping people see oppressive ideals about bodies and seeking greater representation of body diversity in media. Our approach builds off these efforts and echoes what is now known as "body neutrality" or "body acceptance": valuing women for more than beauty, with respect for all bodies regardless of appearance or ability. With those stepping-stones, we seek to provide not only the skills to help you survive and cope in our objectifying environment, but also a treasure trove of skills to radically alter the way you see and relate to this environment, yourself, and everyone else. Rather than helping you feel temporarily good about your appearance, cultivating body image resilience can give you the ability to prioritize your own first-person perspective on your incredible body — regardless of how you look or how you or others feel about your looks. That difference is crucial, because reconnecting with your life's power, purpose, and possibilities outside the framework of looking or feeling beautiful is what will make the difference between adapting to an uncomfortable environment and fighting for a better one.

In our own lives, all the years we spent adapting to our shame and self-objectification by avoiding swimming and trying endlessly to improve our appearances never actually helped us. Even

if we fit into the smaller sizes we dreamed of and others complimented our shrinking bodies or clearer skin or new beauty
choices, we did not feel "fixed." What *did* help was sitting in class-
rooms and reading books and articles that shattered the glass on
our body-centric worldviews and taught us to see more in our
objectifying environment. Learning to see more in the world allowed us to see more in our own body shame—what caused it,
who benefits from us feeling it, and how common it is, regardless
of how we look. Seeing this reality became a catalyst for change
in our lives, but it didn't happen overnight. For years of schooling,
we were able to intellectually understand the ways manipulative
advertising and media messages have warped women's perceptions of their bodies, even as we perceived our own bodies as so
flawed that they were deserving of embarrassment. We knew on
some level that the ideals we were holding ourselves up to were
not innate and natural—they were engineered and designed to
exclude most of us, to push us to hide and fix our endless flaws
forever. But still, they held great power over us.

From Lindsay: I didn't question my allegiance to those unreal
ideals until I faced a familiar disruption, at age twenty-one. It
was the same basic scenario I had faced many times before: being invited to go swimming. This time, it was cliff jumping at a
local reservoir with my wonderful friends and my nice boyfriend.
I had seen pictures from a friend's previous trip, and it looked
awesome, but intense fear and shame knocked me out of my body
image comfort zone at the thought of going. I offered the same
immediate response I always did by making my best excuses to

hide while mentally making plans to fix my body so I could qualify to go next time.

But this time, clinging to my comfort zone didn't soothe me or quiet those negative feelings the disruption stirred in me. I had a different kind of negative feeling in my gut: Sadness. Disappointment. Confusion. Self-betrayal. A thought registered in my mind: *You want to go. Why are you saying you don't want to go? Why are you making these excuses?* I knew the force behind my disruption was body shame. I couldn't even bring myself to defend my flimsy excuses about being too busy when my friends pushed back on them. Without giving a solid answer, I went in my bathroom alone and felt almost panicked about *why* I was considering going and what repercussions that might have for me. Would the old swimsuit in the back of my drawer fit? Would I look so much worse than the other girls going? Would my boyfriend be embarrassed of me? Would he not be attracted to me anymore?

Standing alone in my bathroom, I started to recognize that this disruptive wave of embarrassment about how I looked in a swimsuit didn't have to knock me down or drown me. I chose to actively, intentionally challenge my belief that my appearance disqualified me from going swimming. Rather than letting that wave send me reeling into another fruitless cycle of hiding and fixing, I chose to respond in a new way: head-on.

I quietly worked up the courage to put on a swimsuit, telling no one what a big deal this was for me or how long it had been since I had swum. I sat anxiously in the car on the way to the reservoir, walked behind everyone on the trail toward the water, and watched as everyone grabbed rafts and float toys to help get them across the water to the cliffs on the other side. When they were all distracted, I dropped my towel and waded into the cold water by myself. As it got deeper, I immersed myself in the water and pushed off the bottom, swimming my first strokes in years. I was immediately overwhelmed with the memory of what it felt like to swim, and how exciting but totally natural it felt after six years away.

There in that cold water, alone, I was completely overcome with one of the most deeply empowering feelings I have ever experienced. I was overwhelmed with the feeling that I was still capable. I was okay. My fears about how I looked in my swimsuit immediately washed away, and they stayed away the rest of the day. I was able to see that I had been stuck in an endless loop of trying to fix a body that never needed to be fixed, in order to do something I never stopped being able to do.

When we respond to our disruptions in a new way, seeing more in them and ourselves, they can transform from waves of destruction into waves of opportunity. That same disruption that would always push me to shrink became my opportunity to push back on my shame and grow by tapping into the knowledge and resources to which I already had access. I chose to prepare for the waves and then swim with them, letting them propel me, rather than letting them destroy my makeshift sense of comfort and push me under. And because of that new response, I learned and relearned something I couldn't have discovered any other way — I am still a swimmer. I love swimming. ***My body was never the problem; my perception of my body was the problem.*** My choice to confront a familiar disruption that day in 2007 truly changed my life. Every time I feel tempted to hide or fix, that lesson reminds me that I can just *be* and *do* instead. I don't watch myself live—I live. I rise with body image resilience.

Choosing the path to resilience after a disruption requires an intention to confront shame rather than simply adapt to it and let it be your new normal. I didn't start on the path toward body image resilience because I made one choice to confront my shame; I found it by facing a wave of disruption prompted by an invitation to go swimming and allowing it to work as an opportunity to *see more* and *be more* than a body by leaving behind my uncomfortable comfort zone. To this day, I have never missed out on an opportunity to swim, regardless of the circumstance or who might see me. I have made a new, happier choice again and again, and it has brought so much joy to my life and helped me experience my body as my own.

But this isn't just about swimming. Our own experiences with body shame, insecurity, and self-objectification in our teens and twenties led us to having our hearts and minds opened to the reality of what so many other people experience in a culture that values our bodies first and our humanity second. With that personal experience to fuel our work, we pursued ten straight years of higher education, culminating with earning our master's (2009) and doctoral degrees (2013) at the University of Utah. We founded our organization, Beauty Redefined, in 2009, with a simple blog and Facebook group to share our master's and doctoral research, and have been running a nonprofit by the same name since 2013. Since then, our More Than a Body movement has grown and evolved as we have shared our research on social media, through our online body image resilience course, and by addressing many thousands of people across the United States at live speaking events and reaching millions more online. We never could have found this important work and our shared purpose in helping other people without our own experiences with painful self-objectification and body shame. We also could never have spoken up and showed up in such visible ways — with all the associated criticism faced by women who dare to have bodies and use their voices — without confronting our own self-consciousness and practicing our own ability to rise with body image resilience.

We have put this skill set into practice over and over again in our own lives, but we have also seen it work in the lives of many others. Remember that baseline question we asked our research participants and students in our online course — *How do you feel about your body?* While the majority answered with self-objectifying responses that reflected their negative feelings toward the look of their bodies, about 12 percent of women in our research responded by describing what their bodies could do, the things they had accomplished and experienced with their bodies, and how they felt within their bodies, all without prioritizing an outsider's perspective to simply describe their appearances. Those same women who didn't respond in self-objectifying ways also tended to feel more positively about their bodies.

In digging deeper into the lives of these women in our doctoral research and those of hundreds more girls and women in the years since, we found that many of those who feel positively toward their bodies and do less self-objectifying have also experienced some kind of major disruption to their body images. Those waves of difficulty prompted a significant shift in how they related to their bodies and coped with shame. Experiences included sexual abuse, watching a loved one struggle with an eating disorder or struggling with their own eating issues, teasing or bullying, or experiencing a severe injury or illness that put them on the sidelines of their lives and changed their bodies in unexpected ways. We saw the power of body image resilience through their stories. Instead of clinging to comfort-zone life rafts or sinking into shame in response to their disruptions, or after going through periods of coping in these harmful ways, each of these women was spurred forward to access personal strengths and learn skills to ultimately feel even better about their bodies—not *despite* their pain, but *because* of what they learned while responding to their pain.

The path to rising with resilience isn't an easy one, but it can yield incredible transformations that prove to be well worth the effort of leaving behind our comfort-zone life rafts. Remember the thirteen-year-old-girl in Tennessee who was cutting herself and messaged us about it? That was in 2015, and we are thrilled that her story didn't end there. She wrote to us after attending our presentation, saying, "Like you guys said, I can either use my experiences to make me or break me, and I'm going to use them to make me a stronger, more compassionate person." She reported that she stopped cutting herself, giving us excited updates at twenty-four days and forty-five days with no self-harm and then at months and now years later, saying it had been very difficult, but she was receiving professional help and working to help others with similar pain by being a good friend and spreading uplifting quotes around her school. In 2020, after a couple of years without hearing from her, we reached out to check in. She simply replied, "I'm 18 now and I've been keeping up with you guys. Your messages have changed my life and I've been so much happier." In the absolute depths of sinking into shame, this young girl (now woman) is a shining example of the resilience that is possible not just in spite of our hardest moments, but because of them.

And the girl who wrote to us from her eating disorder treatment center about her attempted suicides? Days after our presentation on body image resilience, she wrote to update us on her situation: "Right before you came to speak to us, my grandfather passed away. My world was ripped into pieces, I fell back into old habits at an alarming rate. In the days leading up and afterwards I had stopped showering, doing my laundry, brushing my teeth, etc. I felt disgusting inside of my skin all over again. When you presented, I was reminded of the hope I had given away. I felt in my heart that your message was true. That evening I took a shower, did my laundry, and brushed my teeth. I also sat down and prayed for an hour straight until my eyes were raw from tears. I prayed with my entire soul, with my entire being. What you said resonated so much with me, and a lot of things suddenly made a little more sense. I will soon be heading home to take my first college class and baby step towards my nursing degree. My purpose is to bring light into this world, not to decorate it."

The painful experiences, beliefs, and feelings that may have kept you sinking into shame or clinging to your uncomfortable comfort zone by hiding and fixing can be your catalyst for positive change. Even when you didn't deserve what you experienced and it is the worst thing you can imagine. When body shame and anxiety rise up, do not turn against yourself to hurt and judge yourself in all the old ways. Don't let those feelings push you into temporary coping strategies that hurt you even more. Instead, look at those waves as opportunities for forward motion to power your venture back to your body as your own. Your body is your home. Your ultimate comfort. Your respite. Yours and no one else's. Look at every disruption to your body image and your relationship to your body as an opportunity to grow and learn and come home with more power and purpose.

Throughout this book, we share the strengths, skills, and tools required for developing body image resilience. Some are innate and natural. Others can be honed through learning and practice. Equipped with the resilience resources you will gather in the chapters to follow, each wave of shame or hurt from objectification you experience can be an opportunity to kick against those pressures and access your skills for becoming embodied and connected with who you really are, and who the world needs you to be.

2

Critiquing and Creating Your Media Environment

- What influences the way you feel about your body?
- Which specific sources, messages, and experiences have shaped the way you think about your own body and others' bodies?

See More in Media

Girls get the message, from very early on, that what's most important is how they look, that their value, their worth depends on that. Boys get the message that this is what's important about girls. We get it from advertising, we get it from films, we get it from television shows, video games — everywhere we look. So no matter what else a woman does, no matter what else her achievements, her value still depends on how she looks.

—Jean Kilbourne, creator of the film series *Killing Us Softly: Advertising's Image of Women*

Mapping Your Body Image

Television, movies, magazines, video games, and social media are some of the most prevalent—and inescapable—sources of messaging that objectifies women and girls, and their reach begins in childhood. Slowly but surely, we piece together each new message we receive to form our very first body image maps, where X marks the spot at the destination of "feel beautiful." These are the maps we will use to understand and navigate the treacherous waters of objectification for years to come. Formed in our minds but as tangible as a handheld document, our body image maps shift and evolve over time based on changing currents of beauty ideals and the discovery of new routes toward body confidence and desirability. The messages and ideas that inform these maps are ever present and inescapable. Assuming you've glanced at a magazine, driven past a billboard, watched TV or movies, or scrolled through Instagram's most popular profiles in the last few years, you've got a good idea of what media's definition of an attractive, healthy, "normal" woman looks like, and it likely shows up in your own body image map. The mold you hope to fit likely looks young; very thin but with curves in all the "right" places; with thick, smooth, shiny hair; full but manicured brows; long lashes; pouty lips; a small nose; and pore-, zit-, cellulite-, and wrinkle-free. If you have light skin, you've got a tan, "healthy glow." If you have dark skin, you're not "too dark."

On Instagram or other social media, the ideal-looking woman

is probably featured in and sharing lots of beauty-focused and body-centric content because she knows exactly how to increase engagement with her brand. People around her often talk about her beauty and attractiveness, and the comments are on fire about her body and fashion choices. In movies or TV shows, she might be relegated to being the love interest or object of desire, or if she does much else, she does it while wearing something outrageously inappropriate for the situation (while the men around her are in fully functional clothes)—defying death with a corset on or running for her life while wearing five-inch heels and a soaking-wet translucent top.

It is no wonder that so many girls' body image maps lead to just a few similar, narrow destinations that just happen to resemble their favorite princesses, pop stars, and influencers. The destinations we think we're looking for are in mostly the same places, like fitting into those jeans in the back of your closet, wearing a bikini proudly, getting your "body back," or ridding yourself of those forehead lines and crow's feet. The routes and shortcuts to get to these destinations vary, from surgical interventions to a full-time commitment to that workout plan or diet, but there is no shortage of options promising you happiness, comfort, love, and success, as long as you stick to the path or pay the right people to guide you.

Our mental images of these dreamy destinations on our maps are shaped by super-cohesive messages that reach us from every angle imaginable. These messages show only a narrow range of acceptable bodies and appearances. If your natural shape and looks fall outside that range, whether just outside the boundaries or what feels like an eternity away, lots of people and companies have charted courses that profess to help you get there — promising that the cost and effort will be more than worth it for the reward of an oasis of confidence and attractiveness at the end.

In media, including social media, children's movies, and even the local news, women are represented far too often as pretty parts served up on a platter. Not thinking, feeling humans, but bodies to be consumed. This sneaky objectification, which literally turns people into parts, happens in children's cartoons when the curvy, long-lashed female animal (*animal!*) is introduced, swinging her hips and catching the eye of her male animal counterparts, and the bow-chicka-wow-wow music starts playing. In the largest study of its kind, the Geena Davis Institute on Gender in Media found that in the top one hundred family films of 2017, male characters outnumbered female characters at a ratio of 2:1 when it came to leads, screen time, and speaking time. Of the female characters that existed, the majority were highly stereotyped and hypersexualized. Startlingly, their 2016 report found that female characters are three times more likely to be shown in sexually revealing clothing than male characters and three times more likely to be verbally objectified than male characters.

Normalized objectification happens in the checkout aisle when a magazine's Woman of the Year is nearly naked on the cover and the Man of the Year is in a full suit and tie (we're side-eyeing you, *GQ*) and when all the headlines on women's magazines revolve around weight loss and beauty enhancement. It happens when male news anchors are allowed — even encouraged — to visibly age, go gray, and embrace their "silver fox" status, while female news anchors sign contracts that require them to maintain their low weight, get producer approval and direction on their hair and clothing, and often undergo anti-aging procedures. It happens when women are cast for movies and TV only when they fit narrowly defined beauty ideals, while men get to represent a wide array of looks and characteristics. It happens every time the camera tilts up and down a woman's body on screen, focusing in on her parts as if the viewer is always a heterosexual male onlooker (and that happens a shocking amount when you pay attention).

Women on screen are much more likely than men to not have speaking roles and to be naked or half naked, and the percentage of female teens depicted nude or seminude has increased dramatically in recent years, according to the New York Film Academy. These stats are then reflected on social media, where engagement increases many times over for girls and women who take off their clothes or post body- and beauty-centric content.

Entertainment media further warps our reality through a double standard in acceptable ages for the men and women on our screens. A whopping 62 percent of women in the US are over forty. But get this: older men appear as much as ten times more frequently than older women in entertainment media. In the highest-grossing films of 2018, 45 percent of male characters were forty and older while only 31 percent of female characters fell in the same age group. Even when film depictions of relationships feature older men, their girlfriends and wives are most often decades younger (see the roles and sometimes the real lives of Johnny Depp, Leonardo DiCaprio, all the James Bonds, and countless more). Men in all forms of media are featured well into their seventies, while women tend to start becoming scarce in media right around age forty. Scholar Gaye Tuchman coined a term for the egregious underrepresentation and stereotypical representations of women: *symbolic annihilation.* Unfortunately, the effects of that annihilation on women's body image, feelings of self-worth, and bank accounts aren't so "symbolic."

With older women being scarce in entertainment media, the way they're represented becomes especially important. Think of the wise, funny, intelligent, "sexy" image represented by leading men well into their fifties, sixties, and seventies — Harrison Ford, Bruce Willis, Denzel Washington, Colin Firth, Javier Bardem, Tom Cruise, Liam Neeson, Jason Statham, Will Smith, George Clooney . . . It isn't hard to think of a list of examples from past or present. In the music industry, male artists enjoy popularity late into their lives, too — just consider who has performed in the wildly popular Super Bowl halftime show over the last twenty years: Paul McCartney, Aerosmith, Bruce Springsteen, Red Hot Chili Peppers, Sting, the Rolling Stones, Lenny Kravitz, the Who. Trying to come up with an equally long and diverse list of female movie stars and music industry equivalents over age fifty is more difficult. Thankfully, there are some women actors who fit this bill, like Meryl Streep, Julia Roberts, Helen Mirren, Viola Davis, Julianne Moore, and Diane Keaton, though few are considered "sexy" and paired alongside a younger partner like their male counterparts. Naming female music artists performing at the Super Bowl halftime show is much more difficult: Madonna and Jennifer Lopez (sliding in at age fifty) are the only two women over fifty who have *ever* performed.

When we were kids growing up in Idaho in the '80s and '90s, we stepped into the shallow waters of objectification and began constructing our own body image maps while watching our favorite show in elementary school, *Saved by the Bell*. Our shared first crush (the first of too many shared crushes, onscreen and off, unfortunately), Zack Morris, always pursued the perky, beautiful Kelly Kapowski and other close variations of her character while audiences pitied the chubby, dorky girls Zack reluctantly had to take out on dates along the way.

From Lexie: After watching a prom-themed episode of *Saved by the Bell* after school in fourth grade, I finished a bath by standing in front of a full-length mirror with a towel wrapped around me like a form-fitting tube dress. I wondered if I would ever get invited to go to a dance, if I would wear something similar, and if I would ever be skinny enough to qualify for either. And it wasn't just *Saved by the Bell* instilling fear in my heart that my body wasn't thin enough — compounding it was every other kid and family show out there in which every single girl or woman had a very thin body — from *Full House* and *Fresh Prince* to *Clarissa Explains It All, California Dreams, The Wonder Years,* and everything in between. The rare exception to this ultra-thin rule was the character Topanga from *Boy Meets World,* who was unarguably stunning, but with ever so slightly more curves than the other TV love interests.

The girls on those shows shaped and reinforced what we were learning about what it means to be a woman — that thinness is paramount, leading women's primary role is looking hot and being pursued by men, and women and girls who aren't conventionally attractive are the funny sidekicks, supportive friends, ghastly villains, or the butt of the jokes, but never qualified to be the star or love interest. I'm not at all surprised I felt too fat to be normal, acceptable, or loved at age nine. If I never saw any other body type represented positively in media, how would I know any different?

It would be a few more years before we were fully immersed in the sea of objectification, but even as young girls we had already begun to sense that to live our best, most fulfilled lives would require us to look a certain way. Those simple experiences, cultivated by innocent-seeming media exposure and the reinforcement of those ideals by well-meaning family and friends commenting on their own bodies and the bodies they valued or devalued, began to distort our body images, making our bodies into something to be seen, not sensed. Our body images moved from a part of our holistic self-perceptions, experienced from inside ourselves, to a separate, external, one-dimensional vision.

Steered by advertisers, the toys we played with, media makers, and even loved ones, we sought body confidence and the kind of thinness and beauty that would make us worthy of love and success — and what we found was almost always *nothing*. A mirage. A lie. We followed those maps as if our lives depended on it, but even our most dutiful attempts at clearing up our skin or buying the coolest name-brand clothes or losing weight didn't yield the results we were promised. Using that face wash advertised to us during Saturday morning cartoons didn't make our faces glow. Those super pricey jeans might have won us a compliment or two, but cooler styles and brands kept coming out and our babysitting and lawn-mowing money couldn't keep up with the demand! The yo-yo dieting we began before puberty yielded short-term weight loss, followed by inevitable weight gain soon after when we couldn't keep up with the life-consuming restriction.

By the end of fifth grade, our best friend was taping pictures of Victoria's Secret models to the back of her bedroom door for weight-loss inspiration. We obsessively gleaned fashion and beauty tips from teen magazines and mail-order fashion catalogs. By age thirteen, we began recording our weight-loss attempts in our diaries.

From Lexie: In one of many entries over the years, I wrote: "I started dieting the Monday after we got back from camp. It's my third day today. I'm doing good! Last year I lost 10 lbs in 12 days. I know I can do it again. I want to weigh [goal number] or less. I won't stop until I do. I am so excited! I'm going to be skinny for school!" This is the sneaky danger of objectification. Instead of spending my summer jumping on our backyard trampoline, camping, and Rollerblading with friends (all things I loved), my joy was wrapped up in the hopeful anticipation that I was shrinking my little-girl body and it would be visible to the other kids at school. My looks, and my hopes about how I could look and how that would change my life by allowing me to be loved and more popular, superseded everything else. And that destination I was hoping to reach was always moving out of sight—I had already proved it! I had lost a dangerous amount of weight in a short period of time as a twelve-year-old, experienced no dramatic life changes other than feeling fainty and obsessive about food, and a year later was now hoping to lose the weight I had gained back.

As we all flounder in the sea of objectification, we pursue idealized destinations of beauty/thinness/happiness that are advertised to us as totally reachable if we just implement simple beauty and "health" solutions, but those destinations always prove to be mirages that move farther and farther into the horizon the closer we get to them. They always seem to require the payment of one more toll, one more purchase to improve our ever-changing beauty tool kit, or one more opportunity to hitch a ride behind someone who says she has *definitely* been to that oasis of effortless beauty and thinness and knows *exactly* how to get there. She probably even has photos to prove it (although you don't know what went on in postproduction of that photo). You want to get there too, but where will the map really lead you and what sacrifices will you have to make along the way?

Most media messages about women's bodies are based on the idea that our happiness, health, power, and relationship status depend upon our consumability—how good we look to others and how irresistibly sexy we are. Media influencers, advertising experts, and major commercial industries sell us these objectifying ideals so consistently that they normalize our discomfort and make most of us feel abnormal and subpar in our natural states. Almost all of the mainstream TV shows and movies we watch feature *only* women who fit the ideals their advertisers are trying to sell. Entire industries—what a character on Marti Noxon's TV series *Dietland* (based on the book by Sarai Walker) refers to as "the dissatisfaction industrial complex" — rely on the foundation that women don't qualify to be seen, desired, and consumed, *unless* we buy the heaven-sent products and services made just for us. Men aren't nearly as frequently defined by these flaws or prescribed their solutions — but wow, did women hit the jackpot! And so did the industries who bank on our allegiance to this lie.

In order to see the power these objectifying messages have in our lives, it is vital to understand the profit-driven nature of media — including social media. Media makers, advertisers, and beauty, fashion, fitness, and diet industry leaders know a secret many of us have not yet figured out: the purchasing power of women is unrivaled. Women control more than $20 trillion in worldwide spending, and 75 percent of women are the primary spenders in their household. The earlier we can be introduced to the sea of objectification and feel at home there, the more profitable these companies and ideals will be. If you can convince a girl that makeup and dress-up kits and princess ideals of tiny noses, chins, and waists along with big eyes and busts are not only preferred but necessary — because her very value is built upon being decorative — you've got her attention and investment for life.

As we critically consider representations of women and girls in media, advertising targeted at us, and how we are so often minimized and manipulated out of reality, these questions become inevitable: Why do media makers insist on representing only certain types of women as beautiful, successful, and worthy of being loved? Why is digital manipulation an industry standard for women but not for men? Why does so much advertising target only women with promises of miraculously ideal bodies, poreless skin, richly colored hair, scar repair, soft skin, fuller lashes, wrinkle-free faces, necks, and hands, and so much more? Why is social media filled with young, thin, heavily made-up "influencers" flooding their feeds with aspirational ideals that always happen to be #sponcon (aka sponsored content)?

The answer to these questions is often about the bottom line: money. Profits are at the heart of much of the dangerous messaging that becomes the wallpaper of our lives. Almost all media outlets and platforms depend on advertising dollars to operate. Everything you see and hear in magazines, TV shows, movies, lots of news, and almost all social media influencer content depends on the profit those outlets generate from advertising. Because of that, the content has to uphold the same ideals as the ads — making them appear normal and attainable — or else advertisers aren't happy. Digitally slimming and emphasizing parts of women's bodies and removing signs of life like pores, cellulite, and wrinkles aren't just casual decisions based on the aesthetic preferences of a few editors — they are profit-driven decisions to create false ideals for us to endlessly chase after.

#Sponcon and Influencers

The ideals we see in magazines and on TV start to appear even more reachable thanks to the tips and tricks shared by our favorite social media influencers — often in seemingly personal, vulnerable, #sponsored testimonials about how waist shapers (a less oppressive-sounding word for corsets), diet shakes, hair gummies, appetite suppressant candy, trendy new workouts, and laxatives adorably termed "flat tummy tea" help them look their very best. These women just so happen to have none of the flaws or issues the products are claiming to fix. Yet even then, they digitally slim and stretch and blur and alter their photos to make themselves look so perfect that their followers just *have to* know how they achieved that look and will buy anything they endorse. We hope everyone knows that the vast majority of those celebs and influencers are simply copying and pasting a caption written for them by companies to sell a product that they've never actually used. But *not* everyone knows. The most vulnerable among us—the youngest, most depressed, most beaten down, and most desperate to be accepted—often do not know.

Now, on top of more obvious sales tactics from celebrities and influencers and straight-up ads embedded in your social media feed that follow you throughout the web based on things you say aloud (!!!) and things you've searched online or texted to a friend, we have regular-seeming people on our friends lists who are also peddling products in more subtle ways. These include "microinfluencers," who have followings from the tens to the low hundreds of thousands, and "nanoinfluencers," the newest lingo for social media users with as few as one thousand followers, who show up in your social media feed with a tip for their favorite shampoo or skin care product and a barely noticeable #ad hashtag buried underneath (and sometimes not disclosed at all). Use of these sneaky ad techniques is growing thanks to research that shows people trust recommendations on products and services from people they know (or feel like they know from social media) more than traditional, obvious advertising.

It is expected that the total advertising dollars spent on influencer marketing will rise from $5 billion in 2019 to $10 billion within the next five years, according to the influencer marketing firm Mediakix. Be on the lookout for how swiftly friends and friends of friends start to see you as a potential customer rather than a social media buddy, and be on the lookout for how you might see your own friends and family that same way. Women are prime targets for this type of unexpected direct marketing via social media, and the types of products being peddled often reflect that. Don't be surprised at how overwhelmingly appearance-centered those advertisements are, whether they are blatantly sponsored posts from celebrities and big influencers, actual advertisements from companies, or subtle shout-outs in regular-looking daily posts from friends. Makeup, hair products, diet and weight-loss plans, fashion items, shapewear, and other body-centric goods dominate social media ads. Keep your eyes out, and you'll see the truth: ***Advertising targeted at girls and women largely relies upon us believing two things: 1) our happiness, health, and ability to be loved are dependent on our appearance; and 2) it is possible to achieve physical ideals — and thus become worthy of happiness, health, and love — with the help of the right products or services.***

Take a moment to consider the products that women sell each other online or in person. How many of them, at their core, rely on women's anxiety about our bodies and beauty in order to drive sales? So many of these products are female centric and focused solely on appearance, though often under the guise of "health" or "being your own boss." Think about all of the requests from sales-based groups, events, private messages, and persuasive posts you've seen just in your own personal life from friends, acquaintances, or even strangers inviting you to buy diet shakes, teeth-whitening toothpaste, body-shrinking wraps and creams, lipstick, leggings, fitness plans, jewelry, makeup, skincare, hair care, anti-aging products, diet and weight-loss plans, beauty-enhancing vitamins, skinny detox tea, or whatever the next greatest product is. You might have even sold some of these products yourself—and we fully understand why you might have done that. However, we all need to be conscious of the sales tactics we have used and with which we are targeted, especially those that rely on "fixing" women's flaws. We are easy prey in a world built upon and reliant upon our literal and figurative buy-in to our own objectification.

Immersed in Objectification from Head to Toe

Ever since each of us dipped a toe into the waters of objectification, we have been using self-critical, objectifying perspectives to view and relate to our own bodies. As women, we are taught to deconstruct ourselves into parts in need of fixing, and every part has several fixes available for the right price. We are asked to be aware of, fix, change, and maintain every inch of our bodies, from the roots of our hair down to the tips of our toes. Starting at the top—literally, at the tops of our heads—let's investigate the media and cultural messages that have shaped the routes on our body image maps in invisible but powerful ways.

HAIR By and large, it is women who are asked to grow out their hair and spend a lifetime caring for its texture, length, color, volume, and style. Black women especially are up against a tremendously sexist and racist disadvantage under this rule. Often required in professional settings to chemically relax or straighten their natural hair or wear a weave or wig, Black women spend undue time and money to perform these ideals and face repercussions for transgressing these rules. Advertising and entertainment media (and the constant conflation of the two) construct and reinforce these hair standards at every turn. Nearly all female TV and movie characters (when represented positively) and countless social media influencers have long, thick, smooth, colored, styled hair with extensions. It's also nearly impossible to be a woman online without seeing advertisements for hair products "because you're worth it" (a profitably inspiring sentiment from L'Oréal). The time, effort, and money we invest in the hair on our heads starts at a young age for girls, and it's a burden many of us bear our whole lives.

Any hair below the scalp is ruled by arbitrary but strict rules about which hair is acceptable, which isn't, and how it should be meticulously maintained or removed. Many of us haven't ever stopped to question or consider the time and energy we've spent on our eyebrows, eyelashes, and body hair removal over the course of our lives. When it comes to eyebrows, many of us know the pain (and eventual numbness) of plucking, waxing, filling, lining, threading, tattooing, and microblading. We can look back and recall (often with a laugh) the eyebrow shapes and misshapes we have succumbed to over the years. (With a dangerous combination of naturally dark, thick brows and late-'90s pencil-thin brow trends, the Kite twins' venture into tweezing at age twelve had lasting repercussions.) The extent of most men's attention to this issue is occasional unibrow cleanup, often at the suggestion of a female partner—no eyebrow-specific gels, pencils, tattoos, procedures, or maintenance required to feel okay stepping out into the world.

What about any hair below your eyes? The message we've gotten since puberty is loud and clear: get rid of it by *any means necessary.* Armpit hair? No. Shave, wax, or laser, and then use Dove's "armpit makeover" deodorant to top it off. From an actual TV commercial by Dove to the female underarms of the world: "You can be a softer, smoother, more beautiful little armpit—you deserve our best care ever, and don't you ever forget that." Hair between your belly button and the tips of your toes? You've got no excuses. Spend a couple thousand dollars lasering it and then repeat that a few more times, wax every few weeks, shave every two days, but don't transgress the ideals of femininity by keeping your natural, protective, hygienic hair no matter how much time, energy, and cash it costs you to remove it. Billions of dollars per year are invested in making sure women uphold these unnatural, prepubescent ideals, and in making sure the totally normal alternative is viewed as unhygienic, unfeminine, and unappealing.

EYES Don't forget your eyelashes! The eyelash-enhancing industry (can you believe there's an eyelash-enhancing industry?) is growing at a rapid rate based on the notion that beautiful women have dark, thick, long, voluminous eyelashes, and —thankfully—we've been offered a million options for achieving this look. False lashes are on trend like never before, moving that beauty work from women onstage or on camera to everyday women in the carpool lane or the office. Sew them in to your regular lashes, use tiny magnets or glue to adhere them, but don't dare to step into the light of day ever again without them or you'll feel as naked as in those "first day of school with no clothes" nightmares you used to have. If you'd rather focus on improving your own naturally growing eyelid hairs, there are a dozen prescription or over-the-counter solutions to growing longer, fuller lashes—just watch out for the side effects of possible blindness or eye color change.

With or without iris discoloration, our actual eyeballs aren't a real concern when it comes to women-only beauty ideals, right? *Wrong.* In 2019, the eye health company Bausch + Lomb released Lumify, an eye-whitening drop marketed exclusively to women with a pastel-blasted TV ad proclaiming, "It is a real game-changer when it comes to beautiful-looking eyes" that makes them look "brighter and more radiant." The lead agency behind its advertising strategy, Blue Chip Marketing Worldwide, described its success positioning the eye drops not as an eye-health product, but as a beauty enhancer, saying, "We positioned Lumify's unique benefits for whiter, brighter, more radiant looking eyes to a new target, the beauty enthusiast . . . Lumify created a 'bridge' between beauty and eye care at retail stores." It's always fun to see new, highly gendered innovations for women's flaws, especially when men have the exact same parts and none of the concerns *or* the pressure to fix them!

SKIN But with all that endless focus on your hair, do not forget about your skin beneath it (as if that's even an option). It's our largest organ, and one that is also a prized commodity co-opted by industries invested in making sure we don't feel worthy of living with it as-is. Consider all the ways you have described your skin "flaws" and had them described to you. Is your skin acne-prone, scarred, rough and bumpy, discolored, too dark, too pale, dry, saggy, drab, lifeless, blotchy, and uneven in tone? Does it have the audacity to have visible pores, stretch marks, veins, moles, freckles, spots, or lines and wrinkles? It likely has most of these qualities, and so does the majority of everyone else's, yet you probably feel abnormal for having them.

The skin on our faces, necks, and hands has been heavily targeted by the anti-aging industry, which rakes in billions of dollars at the expense of women the world over. Women in particular bear the burden of anti-aging ideals. Almost all of our body image maps point to destinations marked by youth. This is no surprise, since aging—for women—is erased and vilified by the anti-aging and beauty industries, which profit in the billions each year at our endlessly aging expense.

We don't regularly see older women represented positively in media, but when we do, by some mysterious magic, they generally fit all of the ideals for young women. Maybe they'll have a few lines around their eyes, but they still have a headline-worthy bikini bod. You can see it at work in countless magazines, billboards, commercials, TV shows, and movies if a woman over fifty is being featured in a positive light or advertising something appearance related. She'll have no lines or wrinkles, tight skin all over, perky breasts, a thin figure, no age or sun spots, and no signs of gray roots or silver strands sparkling through her thick, flowing, richly colored head of hair.

These women have obviously partaken of the fountain of youth, but what did the trick? We've discovered it! Media's age-less older women are often the product of two tricks: digital alteration and cosmetic procedures. Whether we like it or not (and we are culturally conditioned *not* to like it), we start to look different as we age. For men, those changes are most often depicted as normal and even favorable, since looking "distinguished," "rugged," and like a "silver fox" are things we celebrate in them. For women, those changes are to be immediately stopped, reversed, and hidden at all costs. Seriously, *all* costs — financially, timewise, and healthwise. Because you're worth it, remember?

Plastic surgery is the most profitable industry in the US, and Botox is the number one cosmetic treatment. The global anti-aging market alone was worth $42.5 billion in 2018 and is estimated to grow to $55 billion by 2023. Several million people have Botulinum toxin — a neurotoxin that causes paralysis, from the same bacteria that causes botulism — injected into their facial muscles in order to paralyze them and conceal the appearance of wrinkles, a process that must be repeated every three to six months. About 90 percent of the people who get Botox are women. The next most popular procedures are all also for "anti-aging," including soft tissue fillers, hyaluronic acid treatments, and chemical peels.

Women also invest billions at the beauty counter each year in less invasive options to decrease those "fine lines and wrinkles," minimize the look of their pores, and rid themselves of spots that come with age.

Our skin has been claimed not only by the anti-aging industry but also by the tanning and bleaching industries. Did you know that companies like Dove, Nivea, Vaseline, L'Oréal, and Neutrogena sell self-tanners in North America and skin-lightening and -whitening (aka bleaching) products overseas? These companies rake in billions by telling some women that they need "fairer, lighter, whiter" skin and others that they need a "healthy, bronzed glow." These products and their advertising dominate global markets and disproportionately target women. Black women in particular bear the burden of a long history of white supremacy that underlies the pressure to appear more fair skinned.

It doesn't help that the mainstream beauty ideal in the United States has traditionally been—and continues to be—white, making it all the more unattainable for women of color, and especially unattainable for those with darker skin tones. While women like Beyoncé, Jennifer Lopez, Rihanna, Regina Hall, Kerry Washington, Queen Latifah, Tyra Banks, Angela Bassett, Zoe Saldana, Taraji P. Henson, Halle Berry, and others have achieved renown in Hollywood, we've still got a long way to go. When we do see a woman of color represented as a leading lady or beauty icon in media, she often already fits—or is styled, photographed, or Photoshopped to fit—white-centric ideals of having a light skin tone; European features; a thin yet shapely figure; long, straight, thick hair; and all the other ageless, flawless face and body standards.

WEIGHT AND SHAPE One of the indisputable hallmarks of the last several decades' beauty standards is thinness. Dominant body ideals since the 1920s or so have ranged from thin to extremely thin to today's "thin but also curvy in specific areas but still smooth, firm, and flawless." This inescapable, pervasive ideal has been perpetuated by every mainstream media outlet— print, film, and broadcast—and format—entertainment, news, and advertising—since mass media's inception. Women who are anything but thin are routinely, unquestioningly, the butt of jokes, the villains, or the sob story, and very rarely the lead or the love interest (unless the plot revolves around the problem of her weight). This ultra-cohesive messaging about the imperative of thinness and unacceptability of fatness has put immense pressure on girls and women to achieve this look through any means necessary in order to feel not even necessarily beautiful but simply *okay.*

Most people take for granted that thinness is the key to beauty and sex appeal. Yet it is a contemporary social construction— one that has been carefully curated and upheld by industries that depend on our allegiance to this idea. Our inescapable thin ideals aren't simply a naturally occurring, ingrained, universal truth. Here we could cite wide-ranging international beauty ideals, including those in cultures that prize larger body sizes for women that stand in stark contrast to Western ideals. However, it is way too easy for people—especially white people—to wrongfully dismiss those examples as "others," too different from their so-phisticated, modern ways of living and understanding beauty. But we don't even have to look across the world to find alternatives to our modern thin ideals—just look back about one hundred years in the US.

Perhaps the most well-known US beauty icon at the turn of the twentieth century was Lillian Russell, a stage actress and singer born in 1861. Her 1922 *New York Times* obituary repeatedly references her beauty, noting that "for more than 20 years, she had been known as one of the most beautiful women on the American stage." It is believed that at the peak of her fame, Russell weighed approximately two hundred pounds. She was celebrated for her curvaceous figure, as demonstrated in another *Times* article from 1902 about her in which the author extols her "superior beauty." The way she is described genuinely caught us off guard when we first found this reference: "[Russell] is a particularly robust and healthy creature, who takes good care to remain so." Russell's weight, which would be considered "obese" by today's standard (the misleading and ineffective body mass index, which we discuss more starting on page 210), was actually considered a sign of her health and desirability.

Fast-forward one hundred years and the most prominent beauty ideal has dropped about a hundred pounds. British "anti-supermodel" Kate Moss's much-celebrated, extremely thin, "waif" look dominated the fashion industry throughout the '90s and well into the next decade, as she ranked second on Forbes's top-earning model list in 2007 with an estimated $9 million annual salary. Her androgynous frame was lauded by the fashion industry and earned her more than fifty women's magazine covers and high-profile advertising campaigns. Her much-publicized 2009 statement to elite fashion magazine *Women's Wear Daily* that "nothing tastes as good as skinny feels" reflects a dangerous sentiment that continues to pervade women's body ideals while fueling disordered eating everywhere. The dangerous (and blatantly untrue) quote still appears across "thinspiration," or pro–eating disorder, websites worldwide. It is no wonder the majority of women have aspirations to lose weight and girls start mimicking those dieting and restricting behaviors even before elementary school.

Some might be tempted to think the "thick," "voluptuous," or "curvaceous" ideals that have become more popular in the mainstream over the last several years are a step in the right direction —a reprieve from the unhealthy ideals of the past. However, there is no indication that is true. The diet and weight-loss industry raked in $65 billion in 2018 and has grown every year. It thrives even when the economy doesn't. Rates of disordered eating have remained steadily high. Thinness is still an imperative, only now other attributes that aren't typically associated with thinness—large, firm breasts and smooth, rounded bottoms —are also required. That means many girls and women will go to even greater lengths to achieve a look that rarely occurs in nature by surgically altering their bodies in order to shrink some areas and enlarge others.

Aside from fat injections, body contouring, fat freezing, liposuction, breast augmentation, butt implants, and all the other cosmetic procedures on the rise for women, there are plenty of less invasive options being hawked by the celebrities who uphold these ideals. Shapewear or "foundation garments"— girdles, corsets, control-top nylons, and bike shorts—was a $745 million industry in 2019 and is projected to bring in more than $1 billion by 2025, according to market research by Statista. Underlying the success of this industry is the idea that female bodies must be smooth, firm, and shapely with carefully proportioned curves. Whether thick or thin, beauty ideals and trends will continue to ebb and flow like currents and tides, but the specifics don't matter because we are still getting dragged around in the dangerous waters of objectification.

CELLULITE It's everywhere in real life and absolutely nowhere in TV, movies, or magazines. It's unrelated to health, yet constantly depicted as a sure sign of lazy slobbiness. Large or small, the vast majority of women have it, but it gets depicted as shocking headline news in media nonstop. A multimillion-dollar industry has claimed for decades to have the keys to cure it, but it's just as prevalent today as it ever has been. What is this mysterious ailment? Cellulite, of course! In light of current tiny-waist/big-booty beauty standards, one of the most ludicrous expectations for women's bodies is that they be voluptuous yet smooth, free of any "unsightly" lumps and bumps. The very scientific-sounding word for those tiny lumps and bumps, "cellulite," was first introduced into the US lexicon in 1968 by *Vogue* magazine. Before that, it wasn't even considered a problem. Though it shows up on the bodies of at least 80 percent of women (and about 10 percent of men), it has been vilified for decades by industries that profit from our anxiety about any perceived flaws.

Cellulite occurs because of the way women's fat cells attach to skin's connective tissue. No matter how little fat or how much fat they may have, women's fat cells most often attach in a cube-like pattern to skin tissue, which can create the effect of a rough surface. Men's fat cells generally attach in a crisscross pattern that prevents any puckering. To save us from this supposedly embarrassing condition, women are presented with a host of products and procedures ranging from super-invasive surgeries and painful laser treatments to oxygen-depriving and circulation-cutting shapewear and "skin-firming" (and skin-burning!) lotions and potions. The procedures and potions that claim to remove cellulite, and that have the awful before-and-after pictures to "prove" it, have very temporary effects, if any. Many are simply BS. No large-scale study has ever proved the effectiveness of any cellulite-fixing *anything*. Even weight loss does not change the structure or shape of fat cell chambers. That means, regardless of how much or how little fat you have under the surface of your skin, cellulite is inevitable for most of us, and nothing to be ashamed of—regardless of what the tabloids and social media snarkers have to say about stars who dare to show up on the beach with visible dimples on their thighs and bums.

Digital Manipulation

Your ability to see more in media is incomplete without a real understanding of the ways digital manipulation impacts your perceptions of reality. One of the main strategies used to reinforce and normalize a distorted idea of "average" is the overwhelming overrepresentation of extremely thin women who have breast implants, face fillers, nose jobs, and hair extensions—often as an industry standard. On top of requiring women to fit these already unreachable ideals, models, actresses, and popular artists are digitally retouched using photo retouching for print or static images and computer-generated imagery (CGI) for video. On social media, the demanding ideals are ever-more intense, and influencers drive profits and engagement by portraying their bodies as the peak of perfection. It is no stretch to say that digital manipulation is an industry standard that is openly endorsed and defended by media makers and content creators worldwide. Though we hear about digital manipulation controversies all the time and have been speaking up about them for years, media executives and producers consistently use it to an unbelievable extent and vehemently defend it as a perfectly acceptable thing to do.

Our favorite example of Photoshopping comes to us from *Self* magazine's "Body Confidence"(!) issue in September 2009. When superstar singer Kelly Clarkson was digitally slimmed down almost beyond recognition, people noticed. Her appearance on *Good Morning America* within just days of the photo shoot proved that her body did not look anything like the very thin one that appeared on the cover. In her interview inside the shockingly ironic "Body Confidence" issue, Kelly explained how comfortable she felt with her body, saying, "My happy weight changes. Sometimes I eat more; sometimes I play more. I'll be different sizes all the time. When people talk about my weight, I'm like,

'You seem to have a problem with it; I don't. I'm fine!' I've never felt uncomfortable on the red carpet or anything."

Rather than apologizing for the seriously unethical and extreme Photoshopping snafu, *Self*'s then editor, Lucy Danziger, tried to defend her magazine's work: "Yes, of course we do post-production corrections on our images. Photoshopping is an industry standard," she stated. "Kelly Clarkson exudes confidence, and is a great role model for women of all sizes and stages of their life. She works out and is strong and healthy, and our picture shows her confidence and beauty. She literally glows from within. That is the feeling we'd all want to have. We love this cover and we love Kelly Clarkson."

Interestingly, Danziger wasn't satisfied with that statement and felt inspired to take to her personal blog to further rationalize the Photoshopping hack job, writing, "Did we alter her appearance? Only to make her look her personal best . . . But in the sense that Kelly is the picture of confidence, and she truly is, then I think this photo is the truest we have ever put out there on the newsstand."

It's hard to believe anyone's "personal best" is a photo that is manipulated beyond any semblance of reality. They plastered *body confidence!* all over the magazine and quoted Kelly talking about her own real-life, hard-won body acceptance but refused to depict her actual body.

Examples of truly egregious levels of digital manipulation are easy to find in mainstream media and advertising. Seeing that intentional distortion of bodies and faces for yourself can help you spot it on social media, where it's as sneaky and insidious as ever. Consider what digital manipulation as an "industry standard" means in the context of online content creation today. In the twenty-first century, much of the content you are exposed to is in the hands of individuals and their phones, posted on Instagram, Snapchat, YouTube, and the latest social media platforms. It's your friends posting selfies with the perfect amount of Facetune to not be obvious, that fashion blogger you follow who uses an app to stretch her body in some areas and expand it in others while blurring any signs of cellulite, and that influencer who wouldn't be caught on Snapchat or Instagram without a filter and professional-grade lighting. Through normalizing these little steps away from reality, we perpetuate, reinforce, and raise the bar on the body ideals that used to be fed to us—now, we feed them to each other. We're at a point where digital manipulation isn't only a media industry standard, but a personal standard, too.

We see millions more people online than we could ever see face-to-face, and millions more see us through technology in return. Every time we crop and filter and tune our photos out of reality, we distort any sense of normal or natural. It's even more sneaky and dangerous when the unattainable ideals are personally delivered via photos of our friends and favorite celebrities and influencers who are "just like us!" that are presented as normal, everyday life. Though no study could ever be fully conclusive on this front, as many as nine out of ten school-aged girls admit to doctoring their own photos. Skin-smoothing, image-perfecting filters are becoming so common across every platform that even video conferencing systems like Zoom have a "Touch Up My

Appearance" setting. As photo manipulation apps become more ever present, it is imperative to question and consider what you view, what you post, and the consequences of the time you spend submerged in objectifying ideals and trying to emulate them.

From head to toe, we have been trained to understand every part of our bodies as a potential problem to be solved, regardless of how common, natural, and *un*problematic each "problem area" really is. ***None of those supposed flaws would be of concern if we valued those parts of our bodies for the function they serve and how we experience them from inside ourselves.*** All of those supposed flaws and the pressure we feel to fix them are purely the result of evaluating our bodies (and being evaluated) based on how we appear. In this environment of normalized objectification that has colonized every inch of our bodies, we need to shift our attention from being passive objects to active subjects—from questioning how we look to questioning how we've been trained to see ourselves. When you notice that you are divided against yourself, observing and judging parts of your body as if they are objects to be admired, remember that your environment taught you to take on that limiting view.

Be More Media Savvy

> While we cannot directly affect the images, we can drain them of their power. We can turn away from them, look directly at one another ... We can lift ourselves and other women out of the myth.
> —Naomi Wolf, *The Beauty Myth*

As you learn to *see more* in your environment—illuminating the objectifying perspective pushed by profit-driven messages that chart your endless course toward body shame—you gain the ability to deconstruct those faulty beliefs and chart a new course for body image resilience. Your consciousness about the ways your life choices and beliefs about yourself have been warped by outside sources is a game-changer when it comes to reshaping your environment in healthier, happier ways. You are no longer a passive consumer, accepting manipulated messages about your body and worth and enforcing those messages against yourself and others. Your ability to be more savvy and discerning about all the ideas you've taken in—and will continue to take in—will enable you to deconstruct and reconstruct your body image map to better serve yourself and the world that needs you.

The most empowering part of learning to be more media savvy is finding that this is an active—not passive—new way of being. The ability to be media literate and effectively deconstruct your body image map isn't just about knowing what to avoid and how outside messages impact you. It is also about realizing you have the power and opportunity to construct a new understanding of your body and the world you inhabit and experience with your body. You have the power to replace your old, misleading body image map with a new set of skills and resources that can guide you toward resilience. *Your new route requires you to cut out the sources that mislead you and then choose new ways to actively engage, seek, create, innovate, amplify, and contribute to the world of messages that collectively reflect and reinforce your more empowered perspective on your body and your values.*

The Lens of Media Literacy

As your eyes are opened to the skewed, profit-driven messages that have kept you feeling at home in the waters of objectification, you will become much more aware of the lies you've been sold (and maybe bought into) about your body and your worth. What physical or numerical mile markers have you used to determine when you will finally feel happy with your body or allow yourself to participate in a certain activity, be it dating or swimming or running for office or taking that class? Was it a certain dress you used to wear, or maybe never wore but kept as a motivator for weight loss? Or was it a specific weight or number of pounds to lose, maybe a weight you once were or that of a person you hoped to emulate?

Consider all the sources that helped you construct those specific goals or indicators of success and worthiness. You weren't born with those ideas about what would make your body (and you) okay, so take some time to think about where those specific numbers, sizes, and hopes originated. Where did you get those ideas about what would make your body acceptable? Who else do you know who shares these ideas? Has pursuing or reaching your own physical or numerical mile markers brought you the peace, confidence, and happiness you hoped for? Do you like the body image destination you've reached? Would you recommend your path to others you care about?

Back in the '90s, in the years of our journaling our body goals, we would have answered no to those last three questions. However, having our hearts broken by unfulfilled hopes of weight-loss heaven was a great way to become more discerning about our body image beliefs. After years of endlessly fixating on our bodies in attempts to improve our confidence and our lives, we were both caught off guard by the first hints of relief we felt at seeing the unreality of the ideals we were chasing.

At age eighteen, during our first year in college at Utah State University, we took the same Media Smarts class, a required class for journalism students taught by two incredible professors (Hi, Brenda Cooper and Ted Pease!). In it, we were introduced to the concept of media literacy, or the ability to critically question and understand the ways media is engineered to influence our perceptions. Both of our hearts pounded out of our chests as we learned about the ways women's bodies are intentionally represented in limited and idealized ways in TV, movies, music videos, advertising, and magazines due to a combination of sexism and carefully deployed advertising strategies. We both had goosebumps as we learned about the ways our bodies and our sense of self-worth had been warped by objectifying ideals that not only didn't reflect reality, but constructed a new one. Our adrenaline pumped as we considered the time, energy, and money we had wasted in the pursuit of these deceptive mirages we hoped would make us look and feel "normal."

That class marked the first time we were able to see ourselves, our world, and our choices with a new ability to be discerning and critical of what we had believed and taken for granted for so long. We caught a glimpse of what it felt like to critique the ideals and the manipulation behind them instead of critiquing our bodies and our worth.

In that class, at age eighteen, we started the long process of learning how to deconstruct those misleading body image maps that had kept us stranded in the waters of objectification, far from our holistic senses of self. We had been struggling in that environment since middle school, and we had no idea there was life outside of it. Learning the ability to discern between media manipulation and reality reminded us that we had left behind our whole, embodied selves on the shore. That longing for our more-complete identities, unencumbered by the burden of self-objectification and body shame, started to come back, and we felt glimmers of hope that we could return to what we had lost. Over time, we were able to deconstruct and reconstruct our faulty body image beliefs and the ways we viewed our world by looking through the lens of media literacy.

That life-changing introduction to a new way of seeing sparked a flame that has burned through many years of learning and advocacy around body image. With the ability to be informed, critical, and discerning of everything you hear, see, and already believe, you can find relief for yourself and bring it to others. This requires you to educate yourself on the kinds of manipulation at play in subtle and not so subtle messaging about bodies in our environments. These are the kinds of persuasive messages that are designed to spark your mental task list of self-objectification in order to convince you to buy products and services.

Media literacy enables you to challenge your taken-for-granted perspective about bodies and look at related messages in a new way. It equips you to ask the right questions about the messages you're receiving in order to separate fact from fiction so you can see through scammy strategies for supposed body and life improvement. Being a critical media consumer gives you the ability to deconstruct the claims that companies and individuals use to convince you that their products and services are the key to body ideals and confidence, even (and especially) when they don't work as advertised. And they never do—that's why there are new products and services every day and none of them ever stay on the market for all that long or completely take over their industry. We would *all* know if any beauty or weight-loss miracles existed. They don't. So we keep trying and hoping and buying.

Looking at your world through a media literacy lens encourages you to ask critical questions of every message you consume. Are the media and cultural messages in your life real, healthy, in your best interest, or desirable? It sounds really simple, but awareness is a vital first step in the process of taking your power back from manipulative messages.

Jean Kilbourne, author of *So Sexy So Soon: The New Sexualized Childhood and What Parents Can Do to Protect Their Kids,* wrote: "Huge and powerful industries—alcohol, tobacco, junk food, guns, diet—depend upon a media-illiterate population. Indeed they depend upon a population that is disempowered and addicted . . . And we will fight back, using the tools of media education which enable us to understand, analyze, interpret, to expose hidden agendas and manipulation, to bring about constructive change, and to further positive aspects of the media."

From here on out, your job as a discerning consumer is to question everything. Critical questioning is really just a process of prompting you to be aggressively and constantly aware of the forces at play (money, sexism, racism, shame, unquestioned traditions, etc.) that manipulate your thoughts and behaviors. Try out the following questions the next time you're viewing any type of media, whether in your social media feed or on TV, in a movie, or beyond. Refer to them when you are alone or share them aloud with loved ones who could use a prompt to be more discerning about what they take in.

- Do I feel better or worse about myself when I see this? Would the people in my life feel better or worse about themselves after seeing this?
    - *Does it spark body anxiety or feelings of shame?*
    - *Does it cause me to engage in self-comparison?*
- Who profits from me believing this message? Who is advertising here? (Look for ads, commercials, and product placement, and you'll see who is paying the bills for your favorite media messages.)
    - *Does this message seek to profit from my insecurities by selling solutions to fix my "flaws"?*
- What kind of audience is this message trying to target?
- How are women and girls portrayed or represented here?

- *Do they have roles that move the plot forward in a meaningful way?*
- *Are they valued for their talents, words, personality, or character, or just their appearance or sexual appeal?*
- Does it encourage me to fixate on my own or others' appearances?
- Does it promote or reinforce distorted ideals of what bodies and faces should look like — either through digital manipulation or featuring only one body type or "look"?

If you don't like the answers to any or all of the above, or if you recognize ways any media messages might be influencing you negatively, you now have a choice to make. Will you unfollow, mute, unsubscribe, or otherwise limit or avoid consuming this type of content? Which particular sources do you think could be distorting your view of reality and reinforcing a misleading body image map? If you want to minimize the negative effects of media in your life, you can start by turning away from the messages that do not serve you and free up time and space to make more discerning choices about what you take into your mind and heart. Set a goal to eliminate any media choices that distort, misrepresent, objectify, or actively harm you or others. Walk out of theaters, cancel subscriptions, turn those tabloids over in the checkout aisle, find a new TV show to love, unfollow that influencer, mute that friend or colleague. You won't regret the sacrifice, and your willingness to be careful and conscious of the messages you surround yourself with will yield immediate rewards. When it comes to the latest body ideal trends and the hottest solutions to newly identified female flaws, ignorance really is bliss. If you don't know about it, you don't have to feel bad about it.

Of course, there will always be media that is both thoroughly entertaining and thoroughly objectifying. This doesn't have to be an all-or-nothing situation in which you either immerse yourself in problematic media and throw caution to the wind or isolate yourself from all potentially harmful content. If you like keeping up with the latest in pop culture and winding down with a good movie or TV series, you can still do that without disregarding your media literacy lens. Watch with a critical eye tuned into the images and messages that might trigger your body anxiety or self-comparison to idealized bodies, dehumanize or marginalize people (which decreases your empathy for others), or cause any other negative effects.

We — Lindsay and Lexie — take regular opportunities to consciously check in with ourselves about the media we consume. We have both always loved TV and movies (so much so that we got multiple degrees in media studies!), but we're selective about what we watch. We have chosen to forego anything that uses sexual violence purely to titillate viewers, for example by depicting sexual violence in a way that prioritizes an objectified view of the victim's body rather than the perspective of the one being harmed, or that uses the sexual assault of a woman as a plot device to motivate the actions of a sympathetic male character. This happens more often than we can even believe in the twenty-first century. While sexual assault is a terrible reality for all too many people, its depiction in entertainment media often reflects a sexualized outside perspective rather than the dark reality of its effect on a person. Jessica M. Thompson, director of the indie film *The Light of the Moon*, described this in the *Dallas Observer* as the "fetishization of rape" in film, saying, "I think rape culture is getting worse in a way because we're not discussing it. If you film [rape] like a sex scene, then it is glorifying it."

We also work to avoid anything that consistently reduces anyone to an object for others' consumption—not only to reduce our own tendency to self-objectify or self-compare, but also to avoid rage yelling at the screen the whole time. This one is *difficult*, to say the least, and often comes down to doing a little research—for example, on whether any potential nudity or state of undress is reserved solely for the female characters. Having your eyes opened to the manipulation, sexism, racism, double standards, and overwhelmingly female objectification in so much of popular media is both a rewarding way to live and an exasperating one. Watch, listen, and scroll at your own risk.

One helpful device to be more discerning about the status of women in the shows and movies we watch is known as the "Bechdel test," popularized by graphic novelist Alison Bechdel. It is extremely simple and has a couple of variations you can use to serve your needs. Though it doesn't filter out every piece of media that isn't feminist or empowering, it does help illuminate the sad state of women's representation in so much mainstream media. For a movie to pass the Bechdel test:

1. it has to have at least two named women in it;
2. who talk to each other;
3. about something besides a man.

This depressingly low bar doesn't even require that female characters drive the plot forward or have power in any way, but it does illuminate how often women's experiences and perspectives are simply overlooked or diminished. As you put movies and shows you love to the test, you may not be surprised to learn that more than 40 percent of all US films fail miserably, according to researchers at Duke University in 2017. While films are more likely to pass the test today than in the '70s, this research team found that since 1995, *no progress has been made*—that is, the number of films that pass the test has not even budged since the mid-nineties.

Female-driven box-office hits like *Wonder Woman* and *Moana* and *Bridesmaids* are helping convince the movie industry that people are starving for more and for more diverse, nuanced representations of girls and women onscreen. The good news is that ten years ago, only 24 percent of family films (rated G through PG-13) featured females in lead roles, but in 2019, almost half of the top one hundred family movies featured female leads. Progress will continue as the industry actively moves toward gender parity among directors, producers, executives, screenwriters, showrunners, and governing bodies and voting members for all major awards.

Intermittent Media Fasting

Until the whole mainstream media industry deconstructs and reconstructs itself in ways that reflect and value the diversity of human experiences (which might never happen), we can focus on deconstructing and reconstructing our own ideas of what makes us valuable. To do this, we recommend a kind of cleanse. It'll help you get refreshed so you can feel better about your body inside and out and jump-start your healthy choices. It will help you feel so much more balance and self-control so you can feel *A-MA-ZING*. And *this* cleanse is brand new. None of the celebrity health gurus have been selling it, and you'll never see it advertised by any influencers or fitness outlets. And you'll be relieved to know you don't have to drink cayenne pepper juice or buy a pricey supply of juices or forego solid foods and you'll *still* remove countless toxins from your body. But this time, the toxins are in your mind and they're even more harmful to your health.

Those mental toxins have built up from years of taking in distorted, profit-driven messages about what it means to have an acceptable body. This image of what it looks like to be a worthwhile woman, especially, is so ingrained in our cultural wallpaper that we are completely desensitized to it. *This* detox will start to rid you of that numbness so you can move forward with fresh eyes. It's called an intermittent media fast. Rather than cutting out food, you cut out media. You cleanse your mind in order to cleanse your body image.

Choose a time period—three days, a week, a month, or whatever you can feasibly pull off—and avoid media as much as humanly possible. All of it. Do your best not to view or listen to any TV, movies, or magazines or use any social media apps like Instagram, Twitter, Snapchat, TikTok, or Facebook. Even some books, music, and podcasts can be riddled with objectifying body ideals, so cut those ones out. Use your own judgment to determine which options can stay in your routine during your media fast, with an eye on anything that is body centric or selling narratives or products that rely on beauty and weight loss (which probably rules out most things aimed at a specifically female audience).

Without this never-ending stream of biased, profit-driven, idealized, manipulated, filtered, self-promoting messages and images (even well-meaning ones from friends and family), you give your mind the opportunity to become more sensitive to the messages that shape and reinforce your body image map. *Focus instead on what you see, feel, and experience in real life, in your own body, face-to-face with others.*

Intermittently fasting from media will also give you the opportunity to recognize the reasons you turn to media that you might not even be aware of—escape, boredom, avoiding more important things, self-punishment, anxiety, etc. You can see how your life is different and how your feelings toward your own body are affected. You will be better equipped to recognize the messages in mainstream and social media that trigger self-comparison, body anxiety, and other negative feelings. Of our hundreds of online-course participants who joined in a media cleanse as a course challenge, *all of them* indicated they would make plans to change how they use media in order to better support their mental and physical health because of what they experienced when they stepped away. Seeing media messages and their own beliefs with fresh perspective helped them deconstruct those beliefs in ways that better served them.

When you are done with your intermittent media fast, reflect on what you experienced and learned through the following questions. We highly recommend recording your answers and revisiting them when you need a reminder to start your next regularly scheduled fast.

- What did your media fast show you about the role of media in your life? How did you feel? (Be as specific as you can.)
- Looking back on your media use over your lifetime, how do you believe the messages you've been exposed to have affected you? How might those messages have affected your self-esteem or the way you think of yourself?
- Will you make any changes to your media choices in the future because of your experience with this media fast? Why or why not?

In 2013, following a presentation we did for a chapter of the National Charity League in which we challenged the group to try a media cleanse, a sixteen-year-old named Annie emailed us:

"Your presentation left such a strong and powerful impression on me, and I walked into school the next day with a completely different outlook on life. I walked into school thinking about the way I want to be to people, instead of how I simply want to seem to people. Instagram has discouraged me countless times, and I took your challenge to get off of it for the week and I can honestly say I have never felt more liberated. It was

so much easier to be my true self and be content with my life when I stopped comparing myself to the best moments of someone else's deceivingly 'perfect' life. I have been kinder to my family. I have been inspired to take better care of my body. I have been able to focus so much better in my athletics, my school, my LIFE. You really clarified to me how I can be happy ~ by just being myself and seeing the best in others."

In 2018, a professor friend emailed us a glowing essay from one of her students, named Annie — the same Annie we'd heard from five years earlier. She referenced our 2013 presentation, describing how our media cleanse challenge was the first step to deconstructing her distorted worldview and then carefully reconstructing a better one. She wrote:

"I consider the social media fast I did back in the 11th grade as both a milestone and an event of my life. An event can be defined as a potential moment of truth where the world as we once knew it has been shattered. This results in the possibility of a new world forming. During this fast, I remember feeling indescribably elated. I was more in touch with myself than I had been in some time. Perhaps this was due to the fact I was actually living my life through my own senses rather than laying on my bed scrolling through miles of empty posts and updates."

Our dissertation research participants described similar realizations in their one-week media cleanses. One wrote,

"I didn't think I spent that much time online, but I was wrong. I'm in a habit of taking a study break every 10 minutes to check social media, which is not only eating up my time, but it keeps these ideals in my head constantly. I never had any eating disorders or addictions to exercise, but there have been phases when I was worrying way too much about the way I look. I still can't really eat white bread or anything fried or the least bit greasy (even once in a while) without feeling guilty for the rest of the day. I should do a media fast one day a week."

Another said,

"I have never had very high self-esteem or self-worth, and media definitely just makes me feel worse about myself. My media fast taught me that there are far more important things I need to do with my time, and much more fulfilling things as well. The changes I will make when it comes to my media use is to cut back to only getting on my social networks once a day, and then hopefully cut it down to 1–3 times a week."

We recommend practicing this fast regularly (thus its "intermittent" nature), even just one day a week or month to recalibrate after media overload—which takes a toll, whether we notice it or not. Each time you come back to your regular viewing and listening habits, let your expanded consciousness about media's effects in your life—both positive and negative—direct your choices. Watch and scroll through whatever you decide you want to, but do it consciously and deliberately. Cut out what doesn't serve you, and keep what does.

As you learn to regularly, consciously seek out ways to exercise discernment in what you are viewing and taking into your mind, you will be better able to analyze and assess your beliefs about your body and others'. Take time to deliberately question what you see and how it impacts you. Seeing more in your world enables you to see more in your own beliefs and hopes around your body. It will become easier to catch yourself before you get lured into promises of the great things you can qualify for once your body looks like *this* or your food intake and workout regimen look like *that*.

Creating a Better Body Image Environment

Practicing the ability to be conscious and discerning about the body-related messages in your life will help you not only cut out the bad stuff but also amplify and add to the good stuff. In the twenty-first century, we aren't just media consumers—we are media producers. We are producing content that either reflects the waters of objectification and body ideal mirages we're used to or shows people an alternate way to understand their world and themselves.

Use a discerning eye not only on what you expose yourself to in media, but how you represent yourself there, too. Are your camera roll and social media feeds filled with carefully angled, cropped, filtered, or Facetuned images and selfies? Are you capturing and sharing an idealized version of yourself in hopes that others will see you the way you hope to see yourself, somewhere closer to the body ideal you're pursuing? For most of us, the answer is yes.

Turning your critical eye toward your own beliefs and social media presence will help you see more clearly how and why you represent yourself online the way you do, so you can then evaluate whether you are serving up reality or something closer to the ideals you are always trying to achieve. Those little tweaks you make to your photos and videos—the blurring here, the slimming there, the stretching, angling, posing, cropping, and filtering, even the selection of which photos you choose to share (or not share)—influence the way you see yourself every day.

Where did you get the idea that your skin shouldn't have the detail and dimension it has in the original photo or video? Who taught you that your thighs have to have a space in the middle that might not naturally appear? What convinced you that the roundness of your arms or stomach or face or hips needs to be slimmed out? Where did you learn that the smallness in your breasts or backside is a flaw to be stretched and rounded out? The answer to those questions is: the same sources that warped your body image in the first place.

Trying to control or modify the image of yourself that you

share with the world is absolutely to be expected in a world that views and values us as bodies first and people second. But however understandable, it can still be kind of embarrassing to pull back the curtain and look ourselves in the eye when it comes to the ways we represent ourselves online. That glossy version of ourselves represents how we want to be seen, by ourselves and everyone else. It might represent the version of ourselves we hope is just within reach, 10 or 110 pounds and some dedication to toning and cardio away. It might even represent the only version of ourselves we are willing to accept. That ideal, however close or far to our present-day form, might feel like the "real" you, and the body you have now like a temporary problem to be solved.

When you can look your highly curated social media self in the eye and be more discerning about why you value that fantasy version of yourself more than the version staring into the phone in your hands, you can change. You can critique the messages that pointed you to empty mirages of your ideal self rather than your living, breathing, feeling, real-life self. In this process, you might feel drawn to represent yourself on social media differently — to reflect reality and new possibilities for yourself and others who need it. Keep in mind that even regular, everyday people who are posting vacation or family pics get sucked into the pressures to make their posts body centric and uphold certain ideals. If you use social media, whether as an "influencer" or a casual user, and if you're interested in consciously working to step outside the system that values women for their bodies above all else, then we have some tips to help.

Positive–Body Image Playbook for Sharing Socially Conscious Content

Look through your feed and consider your future posts and stories with these guideposts in mind. Your posts pass the test when they:

- Stand alone, without a caption to situate it as "body positive" or "inspiring."
- Avoid disparaging — even jokingly — any body types or characteristics as "flaws" (e.g., *I'm learning to love my thunder thighs* or *I'm so embarrassed/brave to show this pic of my belly rolls*).
- Can't be easily mistaken for #fitspo, #thinspo, or plain old sexual objectification.
- Serve as more than just a #humblebrag or a request for validation about your appearance.
- Advertise only products or services that uphold the values you hope to promote (if applicable).
- Clearly state that they are promotions to sell a product or service if you're making money from it or otherwise benefiting from endorsing it.

If a post doesn't satisfy most or all of the above criteria, consider skipping it or opting for an image or message that does. A good rule of thumb is to consider each of your posts from the perspective of the most vulnerable person in your friends list or potential viewer — like the girl who is struggling with an eating disorder or self-harm who is ashamed of a body that is less "ideal" looking than yours (and is crushed by your comments about trying to lose weight before summer), or like the woman who shares your body type or skin condition or hair texture and is too self-conscious to leave her house without extreme measures to cover/hide/style/fix it (and would be emboldened by seeing you represent your reality without apology or announcement of your bravery).

As you reconstruct your ideas of what makes you worthy and successful, the fleeting validation from others in response to your photos will hold less weight than it used to. You might even start sharing fewer images of yourself and more images of what you're seeing and experiencing, or instead sharing snapshots and stories of yourself doing and being outside the confines of looking how you hope to be seen.

Creating an environment that is less body centric and that welcomes body diversity rather than perpetuating the stress of striving for one perfect look will bring freedom and relief. What else is there to see, experience, and understand about your world and yourself if you aren't held back by self-objectification and shame? While media use is a perfectly good way to connect and disconnect and be entertained, you may find new energy in connecting, engaging, creating, and learning away from screens. You might find the drive to volunteer or gain skills and employment in content creation that puts you in a position of power to make positive change in media—change that can affect the body image environment shared by your communities and beyond.

In that process of rebuilding what you want to see, it is necessary to carefully and consciously replace the misleading messages from your old body image map with new messages, ideas, mantras, and entertainment. Use your media literacy lens to do regular critical questioning of what you find, to measure new options against the Bechdel Test or your own version of it to increase positive representations of women, and to implement regular media cleanses to rid yourself of ideals and ideas that prey on your shame, incite your insecurities, and profit from your loss.

Once you unfollow, unsubscribe, mute, and opt out of those media choices that send you on dangerous, expensive, unfulfilling excursions, you've got a lot more room on your map and time in your day to chart a new course. What do you want to learn or experience? What accounts, shows, books, podcasts, pages, websites, music, and people do you want to listen to? What messages help remind you of your worth and power beyond your body? What inspires you to be more? What expands your vision, your hope, your knowledge and skills? What lights you up and motivates you?

As you actively seek out media that inspires you to be more, you will find that your body image environment will reveal new ways of living, doing, and being that lead to even more fulfilling destinations that have nothing to do with how you look when you arrive. The waters of objectification and the body ideal mirages you've been straining to reach don't have to be your unquestioned reality anymore, but they can provide motivation for you to see more and be more than the limits they have imposed on you.

Helping Kids Navigate Objectification

Kids today are being invited into the waters of objectification younger than ever. If you are a parent, caregiver, or anyone who is concerned about helping children develop a healthy body image, remember that your ability to be both discerning and vulnerable with kids is crucial. They need to know that this body image stuff is tough, and that media makes it really hard for both kids and adults. Take opportunities to be with the kids in your life as they are watching TV, movies, Instagram stories, and YouTubers, or playing video games. Help guide them toward positive choices, including diversity in character size, shape, ethnicity, race, gender, and sexuality, and toward messages that help them identify with people who are different from them. This builds empathy and understanding. It yields compassion and consideration for others regardless of how they look and what ideals they do or do not fit.

Ask them the same critical questions you ask yourself when you're watching any type of media—questions like: Why do these people or characters look the way they do? Do any of them look like me or people I know? Did the people who created this show value girls and women as more than pretty decorations or romantic partners? Is somebody hoping we'll buy something after we watch, read, or listen to this message? How does this message make you feel? How do you think it would make other people feel?

As you tailor these types of questions for the children in your life, you help them learn to critically analyze media as a construction of reality—not reality itself—an ability that will serve them their whole lives. As they pay attention to how they feel and what they are being sold, you can help them learn to curate their media exposure in active rather than passive ways. They can take notes and make lists of what shows are annoying or make them feel self-conscious or don't represent their reality in honest or happy ways and then plan exactly what they want to consume and create. Encourage them to draw characters they'd like to see, to bring them to life with paint, pencils, or electronic drawing or design tools. Help them act out new scenes and stories for these characters to expand their imaginations and creativity.

One of the greatest challenges we all face is how to navigate social media without drowning in self-comparison, objectification, and the insatiable desire for validation. Kids need to be spared from facing these challenges for as long as possible. Anyone who interacts with children knows that every child is different, which makes it difficult to set blanket rules for what age is appropriate for them to have access to social media. We recommend that you err on the side of caution by shielding kids from their own independent social media access for as long as possible. We don't think any kid under age twelve should have unfettered internet access, let alone free range on social media with their own accounts. Even after age twelve, web access should be monitored, restricted, and lovingly guided as much as possible. Use your own judgment as a cautious, caring caregiver, and be open about your reasoning. This will not make you a popular parent or caregiver, but it is the kindest thing you can do for a kid who does not understand what they're asking for. They might think that by not having their own social media profile, they are missing out on the fun things all their friends are experiencing, but what they are really missing out on is often heartache, disappointment, comparison, loneliness, and feelings of inadequacy.

When your child comes to you asking to join one of these photo- and video-driven social media platforms, take the opportunity to talk with them about what research and real-life experience brings to light with a pros and cons list. First, ask them why they want to use Instagram, TikTok, Snapchat, or whatever the newest apps and platforms are. What do they think they will like about it? Listen to their thoughts and consider them along with other things we know people appreciate about social media, like these:

Pros

- You will be able to interact with your friends online.
- You won't be left out of what is happening online.
- You will be able to participate in fun and entertaining communities where people share their talents and hobbies.
- You will be exposed to interesting content and important ideas and people you might not see otherwise, like body positivity, activism for important causes, experts in cool subjects, and people doing good in the world.
- You'll be able to express yourself through posting pictures, videos, and captions.

Next, ask your child to consider what they might *not* like about using the app or platform they are hoping to join. What can they imagine finding or experiencing that could be negative or hurtful to themselves or others? In addition to any ideas they have, take the opportunity to talk to them frankly about what research has shown about how these technologies affect people. Have you seen any of these negative effects in your own life or in the lives of people you and your children know and love? Tell them that. Open your heart and express your love and concern for them in addition to your trust and confidence in them. As appropriate, discuss downsides like these:

Cons

- You might be more likely to experience increased loneliness. Social media can be isolating and leads to feelings of FOMO, or "fear of missing out." While you might like the interaction from likes, follows, and DMs, in the long run, many people are left feeling more alone and isolated.
- You might be more likely to experience depression and anxiety, and the more time you spend on social media, the worse these feelings can get.
- You might be more likely to compare yourself to the people you see on Instagram. Self-comparison causes you to feel less love toward and unity with those you are comparing yourself to. It also makes you feel worse about yourself, even if you think you "win" the comparison.

- You might be more likely to be preoccupied with your looks (also known as self-objectification). Your appearance will be front and center in your mind, and that makes it hard to focus on anything else, whether you like the way you look or not. This can hurt your schoolwork, your relationships, your health, your mental and physical capabilities, and your happiness.
- You might be more likely to experience negative body image, or feel bad about your body, because you will be more sensitive to how you appear after seeing so many idealized photos, ads, and highlight reels.
- You will be more likely to be exposed to harmful messages and ideas and images that you might not see otherwise and might not be prepared to understand, like objectification, pornography, self-harm, pro-anorexia ("pro-ana") messaging, digital manipulation of photos, misleading advertising, and beauty represented in very narrow, unattainable ways.
- You will be more likely to become desensitized to the messages that hurt you and that cause you to think about your body and your looks more than who you are as a person, which can lead to feeling ashamed and fixated on your body.

If you decide together that your child is ready to join these types of social media platforms, or if they insist on doing so with or without your permission or knowledge, you can equip them with a few important guidelines that will make a world of difference for their health and safety:

1. Make your profile private and *never* allow anyone to follow you who you don't know and interact with in real life, no matter how they look or how many followers they have, even if people you know follow them.

2. Turn off push notifications. They interrupt your life and steal your attention from much better things, and they are almost never notifying you of anything important or urgent.

3. Avoid the explore page on Instagram or similar features on other platforms. These sites that aggregate public content allow users access to any public post, and they mold the advertised posts to users' interests and what advertisers want to show them, which is often body focused, looks oriented, and objectifying.

4. Set boundaries and time limits. Spend only X minutes on each platform each day, at certain times of day, rather than go back to it constantly and unconsciously. Social media can absolutely be addictive, and the platforms are designed to hook users by providing a rush of satisfaction with every notification and update of new content.

5. Don't allow direct messages from people you aren't already following, and never click on links that are messaged to you from people you don't know or don't know well.

6. Never send nude pictures (of yourself or anyone else) via any app or messaging service. Delete them if you receive them. You could be charged with a serious crime, even for just sharing an image you received from someone

else. These images are almost always used to degrade and humiliate people, and you want no part in that.

Actively Engaging as Consumers and Creators

For the first decades of mass media's existence, radio and TV came into our homes without any way for us to interact with it. It was strictly one-way communication: sender to receivers; media maker to consumers. The internet enabled two major changes to that longtime formula. First, lots of people can now produce their own media messages and reach lots of other people. And second, we all now have the ability to talk back and challenge media messages in public ways through social media. Unlike letter-writing campaigns, phone calls, or even petitions to call for change — all of which can be outright ignored — public tweets and shareable images and posts have provoked significant attention and meaningful responses.

You have the opportunity to participate in shaping what comes into your home and social media feeds, and you have the right to speak up when something is causing harm. Be brave in calling out messages that are hurtful and degrading. Hold media makers accountable for their content and its impact on consumers. Raise warning flags for passersby that these ideals are unsafe and unreachable and that the routes toward them are filled with danger. You might discover you have insights people are eager to hear and amplify.

You can speak up, publicly and passionately. Thousands of

people turn to social media to share their stories of discrimination, prejudice, and pain. They are using their voices and their platforms to call out oppression and mobilize others to help propel change. Being an activist can feel like something reserved for the most privileged among us—those who have a voice people will listen to, the energy and bravery and time to use that voice, and the means to get involved—but it can't be reserved for the privileged alone.

Reframe how you think about activism to make it a part of your life that is accessible and invigorating. It can be as simple as posting or reposting on social media a story about discrimination or injustice or objectification with your own comments about why it matters; agreeing to speak with a journalist or podcaster who is interrogating a topic; exploring these topics academically and professionally; creating art that reflects your experiences or helps illuminate the plight of those who are marginalized; volunteering for an organization that is committed to eradicating injustice; donating time or money to causes you care about and encouraging others to do so, too; marching for causes you care about; and so much more. You can propel change by being an advocate for yourself and others in every way you can. If you are in a position of power, you can use your power to keep someone else afloat. Listen to people and amplify the voices of the voiceless or marginalized in every way you can.

Over the past several years, we and our online allies have waged and won several battles against harmful messages using social media. We joined eating disorder experts, activists, and celebrities like Jameela Jamil of NBC's *The Good Place* in calling out

Kim Kardashian in 2018 when she became a spokesperson for appetite suppressant lollipops. She and her sisters (and hundreds of other social media influencers) promote the same products every day of the year with little to no pushback, but the collective call to action made international headlines. Whether or not reality stars and influencers stop hawking products like these, millions of people were able to catch a glimpse of reality when body image advocates publicly flagged the absolute lie that lollipops or detox teas or diet shakes could make anyone's body look like the Photoshopped creations we see online. In 2019, Instagram established a new rule, blocking Instagram users under age eighteen from seeing posts promoting certain types of cosmetic surgery and diet products. This was a huge win, propelled by Jamil and many powerful activists and scholars on the platform whose voices were amplified all the way up to Instagram headquarters by millions of people.

Also in 2019, dietitians, activists, and experts fired back at WW, the company formerly known as Weight Watchers, when they launched "Kurbo by WW," an app intended to track food consumption, physical activity, and weight loss in kids as young as eight. The firestorm of rebuttals and callouts aimed at WW, including the viral #wakeupweightwatchers hashtag that flooded Instagram and Facebook, was fierce and nearly impossible to ignore across all forms of social media. Natalie Muth, a pediatrician and a spokesperson for the American Academy of Pediatrics, told the *Atlantic* in August 2019 that she is wary of the potential for a tool like Kurbo to turn dangerous in the hands of kids. "Children are not 'little adults,' and the approaches that may 'work' for adults, such as weight-loss goals, are not appropriate for children most of the time," she said. "Interventions that focus on weight as the main target can trigger disordered eating patterns, low confidence and self-esteem when goals are not met, and an unhealthy preoccupation with looking a certain way." WW proceeded with the app's debut, but it is likely that the fierce public response dissuaded some would-be users.

Mattel debuted a line of body-diverse Barbie dolls because of pressure from online activism. Google has stopped all porn ads and prohibits ads from linking to sexually explicit websites. Target is including children with disabilities and more diverse models in its advertising after facing public backlash for Photoshopping bikini models in extremely irresponsible ways. After years of harmful messaging thriving in the dark corners of social media, almost all of the big media platforms are working to make sure that certain pro–eating disorder and self-harm hashtags are not only unsearchable, but lead to a message that urges people who need it to reach out to the National Eating Disorder Association and other professional help—all thanks to social media activism. To express solidarity with others who have faced sexual abuse and assault, activist Tarana Burke coined the simple phrase "Me Too." In 2007, she started her own nonprofit to support victims, and in 2017, following sexual abuse allegations against Hollywood producer and convicted rapist Harvey Weinstein, that phrase set off a massive movement and became a hashtag that millions of people mobilized around. The impact of this online activism continues to be felt throughout the world as women are encouraged and empowered to share their experiences and seek justice.

With social media, your voice can make a greater difference than ever before. Being more discerning and careful about the messages that make up your body image environment is a foundational, transformational strategy that will help you rise with body image resilience. Your ability to be more media savvy opens up the possibilities of your own power and potential to be an active, critical consumer and producer—not a passive audience—and to use, create, and enjoy media in a healthier, more empowering way.

3

From Self-Objectification to Self-Actualization

- Have you ever stayed home or not participated in an activity, sport, event, social engagement, or other opportunity because of concern about how you looked? If so, describe what situation(s) you avoided or opted out of.
- Why did you make that choice? What feelings or fears prompted you to stay home or opt out?

See More in Yourself

Men act and women appear. Men look at women. Women watch themselves being looked at. This determines not only most relations between men and women but also the relation of women to themselves. The surveyor of woman in herself is male: the surveyed female.

Thus she turns herself into an object.

—John Berger, *Ways of Seeing*

As self-objectification creeps into your life, your identity is split in two. Instead of your whole, embodied, thinking, feeling self, you become a distant observer. During a lunch meeting with a coworker, you find yourself being interrupted by your worries about holding in your stomach, whether your coworker will notice you lost or gained weight, how your body looks in your chair to the people sitting behind you, and whether this lighting is doing you any favors. You schedule an hour to hit the gym, and as you are on the treadmill, you become distracted by what you look like in the mirror facing you as you tug and adjust your clothing, and wonder what the person on the machine behind you is seeing as you run. You are detached and self-conscious during intimate moments with your partner rather than being present and passionate, regardless of how positive or enthusiastic they are about you. You slip outside yourself, observing your body from afar countless times each day. Sound familiar? This mental picturing leads to constant evaluation and monitoring of your body, in which you prioritize an outside perspective of yourself rather than your own first-person perspective from the inside. It leaves you disconnected from your own joy, pleasure, focus, full capabilities, and fulfillment.

In 1952, the scholar Simone de Beauvoir described this concept by saying that as a girl grows up, "she is doubled; instead of coinciding exactly with herself, she also exists outside." Social psychologists Barbara Fredrickson and Tomi-Ann Roberts first named this concept "self-objectification" in the late '90s, which they defined as "the tendency to perceive one's body according to externally perceivable traits (i.e., how it appears) instead of internal traits (i.e., what it can do)." This phenomenon mostly affects girls and women, regardless of age and background. ***Self-objectification is the invisible prison of picturing yourself being looked at instead of just fully living.*** It is the soul-sucking act of policing and monitoring yourself against your worst fears of what someone else might be thinking when they look at you.

As your identity splits, self-objectification hinders your ability to self-actualize, or realize your full potential. This dual identity is a burden, a constant distraction, a huge discomfort, and a real limitation to your progress, potential, and happiness. If you think back to our metaphor of existing in a sea of objectification, self-objectification is like wearing a pair of heavy, soaking wet jeans while trying to swim.

The Burden of Self-Objectification

For most of us, paddling along in this waterlogged denim is the default. It's objectively awful, but it's your normal. And even though you're so used to the feeling of wearing heavy, soaked jeans that you don't really question it, they're still holding you back in measurable ways. They make it hard to swim, tread water, float, row, stretch, pull yourself into a life raft, concentrate on anything or anyone, comfortably relax, get dry in a reasonable amount of time — anything, really. The wet denim of self-objectification holds you back literally and figuratively by placing an invisible burden on your mind and self-perception. A portion of your valuable energy is always being dedicated to dealing with that heavy layer of distraction. And there are reasons every community pool has a sign that says, NO JEANS. NO CUTOFFS. They're not only impractical and uncomfortable; they're unsafe — a drowning disaster waiting to happen.

Have you ever tried to run or lift weights or take a reading comprehension test, math test, or spatial skills test while wearing soaking wet jeans? Probably not, but try to imagine it. You most likely wouldn't do as well in any of those areas as you would have without the wet jeans. The same is true for real-life self-objectification — women have been shown to perform worse on all of those tests and activities when they're distracted by or self-conscious about how they look, even if they're alone in a room in some cases.

One of the most insidious consequences of self-objectification is that it fragments our consciousness, disrupting or even preventing us from reaching peak motivational states, or a state of "flow," as it is termed in positive psychology. Flow is a mental state in which you are fully immersed in a feeling of energized focus, full involvement, and enjoyment in an activity. If you've ever been fully absorbed in a task and lost that "doubling" of your identity that self-conscious body monitoring demands, you've known a state of flow. It happens when you are concentrating, creating, moving, writing, and living outside your fears of being looked at. Research shows us that constant attention to physical appearance saps your mental and physical energy, making it nearly impossible to reach or maintain a flow state. Research points to the fact that, as early as grade school, girls' activities and thoughts are more frequently disrupted by critical self-aware-ness and self-consciousness than boys'. Your quality of life and well-being are at stake when your identity is split in two.

What are you — and the world — missing out on because the soul-sucking posture of self-objectification keeps you from doing, being, experiencing, contributing, and achieving in every area of your life? When you live as the surveyor and the surveyed, the watcher and the watched, you come to believe that you *are* your body and you are defined by your looks. You then evaluate yourself accordingly. This generally starts around puberty (although it can start even younger), when you begin to experience what it feels like to be sexualized and objectified by other people, whether that be through lewd comments made by others or your parents insisting you wear a cardigan over your favorite dress or cover up immediately after swimming.

We begin to be preoccupied with our looks, our clothing, our appeal to onlookers whether we're actually being looked at or not. Over time, that passive, appearance-obsessed state starts to pres-ent itself as a mental task list — an ongoing stream of thoughts that remind us to pull up our pants so no belly rolls are visible, cross our legs when sitting in those chairs so our thighs appear thinner, suck our stomachs in, keep our chins up (not in pride, just double-chin patrol), hold our arms away from our bodies to make them look less round, blot our oily faces, and tame unruly hair. Even when we are alone, we body check our appearance in the car mirror, our cell phone camera, or the store window's reflection, or otherwise simply *picture* ourselves living instead of just living.

It is incredibly difficult to feel positively about our bodies if we are judging them only on looks, especially in light of the ideals we're up against. That is truly the root of negative body image. We saw this in the answers women gave to our simple baseline question in our research, "How do you feel about your body?" The vast majority of the women answered that question by describing what their bodies *look* like—the way they *think* their bodies look to others—in mostly negative, appearance-based terms. They said things like:

"I have always been really thin and regularly get told to 'eat a hamburger' to gain weight. People mock me and tell me I must have an eating disorder and it makes me hate my body."

"I feel like I'm too fat or not skinny enough for the world today. I feel like I'm not good enough for my husband because of my body."

"It has never looked how I want it to. There is cellulite, scars, veins . . . things I try hard to keep hidden. I always think, 'Why can't I look like her?'"

We know that when we do not believe we fit the beauty ideals we think we should, body monitoring often leaves us incapable or unmotivated to perform in other areas of life. In all, 71 percent of the women ages eighteen to thirty-five who participated in our doctoral research very clearly self-objectified without even knowing it. But among those who felt negatively about their bodies, that number soared to 91 percent. And based on the self-reported information of participants in our online body image course, 82.5 percent of women stay home from events or activities, or sit out of opportunities, because of their appearance anxiety. That statistic—eight out of ten women—tells us too many women live in a near-constant state of body monitoring.

Our own research and that of so many others illuminate the true tragedy of self-objectification among all ages, ethnicities, and backgrounds, resulting in a predictable set of experiences —negative body image, preoccupation with appearance, disruption of mental and physical performance, shame, anxiety, and depression—and means for coping—disordered eating, self-harm, substance abuse, decreased sexual assertiveness (including not saying no when you want to and not discussing or using contraception), physical inactivity, perpetual dieting, and more ways we "hide" and "fix." When we live our lives in this perpetual state of body monitoring, we are living passively, being judged and consumed by ourselves and others—not as self-actualized humans actively making choices.

In these conditions, we stop raising our hands in class and speaking up at board meetings. We sit on poolside lounge chairs, fully clothed and overheating, while our kids beg us to hop in the water with them. We opt out of the gym, sports, or PE class because we don't want to get sweaty or red faced or be seen in an uncontrolled state of movement. We skip parties, put off running errands, delay family pictures and reunions, and hide at home because of our weight, acne, unshaved legs, or clothes that aren't quite right or because we don't have the time, money, or energy to put on makeup or style our hair.

> What joyful, powerful experiences are you giving up in
> the process of trying to preserve your not-so-comfort-

able comfort zone? Are you held back from progress, happiness, health, fulfilling relationships, and contributing good to the world because of your deep-seated fears of being looked at? Many respondents in our doctoral research were struck by learning about self-objectification and realizing how it had consumed their time and energy:

"Because of self-objectification, I completely lack confidence in my appearance. Although I know I'm a beautiful person on the inside, with a lot to offer to those around me, I still have a very hard time believing I'm beautiful. I find myself hiding behind my clothes. I also never go swimming, even though I LOVE the water, because that would mean I would have to show myself to others in a swimsuit."

"I honestly never even noticed what I was doing until now. I focus on the way my thighs have grown, stretch marks, my 'muffin top.' I notice my breasts may not look the way I want them to. Even my belly button isn't cute. My butt is too flabby and big. My hair is too flat, too ruined. I hate my freckles most of the time. My nose. My eyebrows. I literally have pieces of myself that I pick at. Even my toes. This is so weird for me to think about and even admit to anyone . . . I certainly hide all of the time. I hide from old friends that I want to see so badly because I don't want them to see the 'fat' me. I feel like self-objectification has ruined me."

"I do everything I possibly can to hide my post-baby belly and breasts. I break myself into bits and pieces every time I look in a mirror. 'These should be higher, this should be flatter, these shouldn't even be here, etc.' Between postpartum depression and self-objectification, my life and marriage have been greatly impacted. I very rarely want to be intimate with my husband and will only do so in the dark. I end up in a terrible mood any time I have to go clothes shopping."

"Self-objectification takes a HUGE toll on my life! The focus on my body consumes my thoughts every day! I hide body parts with baggy clothes and padded bras and also want to take extreme measures to fix them. I feel very cranky when I wear pants that make my 'spare tire' show a little. It consumes my life and determines my mood. I have ALWAYS, for as long as I can remember, hated the way I look. I have struggled socially and academically and now I'm thinking that's why—because I have never liked the way my body looks. I desperately want a boob job so that I feel comfortable in the bedroom with my husband, who is also my best friend and says NOTHING negative about my body."

"I have self-objectified my whole life and it's taken a huge toll. I am constantly on alert about my weight and how other people may perceive me. I have tried to hide interest in people that I might find attractive because I think they would reject me anyway. I stay away from getting in pictures as much as possible when I feel

overweight and miss out on capturing a lot of memories. I also fail to make memories, by keeping myself 'safe' from embarrassment or ridicule and avoiding activities. It has caused a lot of anxiety, discouragement, self-loathing, wasted money and time (searching for solutions), shrinking from social situations, and a general feeling of missing out and having life pass me by."

"Junior year of high school I mostly didn't even go to school. I felt ugly compared to the other girls and I hated getting dressed when I felt like I had no clothes to wear."

"I have to gather all my courage and thoughts and just get out there and live life. It takes so much time that I sometimes end up running out of time to go to the pool. Similar things happen when it comes to getting ready for an activity that I feel I need to look a certain way for . . . it can take me a lot of time/frustration to finally get to a frame of thought where I finally just give up to the way I am and look because 'there's not much I can do about it' and I know it shouldn't stop me."

"I avoid swimming, which is a shame 'cause my kids love to swim. I'll wear a bathing suit in front of my mom or sister but avoid being in one in front of my husband, his family, and my sisters-in-law. I've thought about staying home from my husband's work functions because I'm afraid I'll embarrass him. He's very fit and good-looking and I'm always worried people will see us together and think, 'Really? He's with her?'"

In our own lives, self-objectification began to creep in all the way back in elementary school, when during reading time we began comparing the size of our thighs to our friends'—a memory Lexie remembers very clearly as she sat kneeling on the floor in second grade in her stretchy floral shorts. When you can remember an early, specific moment of self-consciousness about your appearance or clear memories of monitoring your body, you should think of those experiences as waves of disruption to your body image that mark instances when you were knocked out of your comfort zone and prompted to respond. Your response might have been a new, diligent awareness of how you appeared and how others saw you, which felt like a natural protective instinct to make sure you didn't look bad or embarrassing.

From Lindsay: I have a clear memory from age eight of coming home after nightly swim-team practice and standing in front of a full-length bedroom mirror. I noticed a dimple in the side of my little thigh and felt sinking shame because of it. I remember thinking to myself, "If I can just keep my hand over this dimple while I'm on deck at practice and swim meets, no one will know it's there and I can keep going to swimming." Without even knowing the word *cellulite,* self-objectification was teaching me to double my identity and monitor myself as if I were my own overseer. That thought became more ever present and powerful as the years went on and our attempts to hide and fix our bodies weren't yielding the results we had hoped they would.

From Lexie: At age fourteen, I wrote in my journal: "I am at one full week of dieting today. I've done a good job. By this time next week I will have lost 10 pounds. I've been very stressed lately. I feel like there isn't enough time to lose weight before swim team starts. I feel like there isn't enough time to get in shape before swim team starts. I feel like there isn't enough time to get a new suit before swim team starts." Later that year, instead of confronting and dealing with my fears of being looked at on deck (after all, "lose weight," "get in shape," and "get a new suit" were all just descriptors for how I thought I appeared to onlookers), I quit the team. I faced the body image disruption of worrying how I looked while swimming by clinging to my comfort zone. Within about a year, Lindsay followed. Neither of us could stand the thought of being seen in our swimsuits, despite swimming being a joyful, empowering part of our lives. We silently vowed to hide from swimming until we qualified to be seen in swimsuits again by "fixing" our embarrassing bodies.

In 2011, author Autumn Whitefield-Madrano started noticing the negative effects of her own fixation on her appearance. She decided to undertake an incredible experiment: a monthlong break from mirrors to liberate herself from self-surveillance, with the goal of achieving better access to a flow state. She had been shaken by a passage from John Berger's 1972 book that shook us equally when we first read it:

> A woman must continually watch herself. She is almost
> continually accompanied by her own image of herself.
> Whilst she is walking across a room or whilst she is weep-

ing at the death of her father, she can scarcely avoid en-
visaging herself walking or weeping . . . And so she comes
to consider the *surveyor* and the *surveyed* within her as the
two constituent yet always distinct elements of her identity
as a woman . . . Thus she turns herself into an object—and
most particularly an object of vision: a sight.

And so Whitefield-Madrano undertook a fast consisting of thirty-one days of no mirrors, store windows, or any other reflective surfaces she might normally use to body check.

While she reported that nothing visibly earth-shattering changed, she became more in tune with herself, her needs, and the "beauty work" she had grown so accustomed to performing (hold my head at this angle, nod and smile, be pretty). And the greater victory: decreased self-consciousness. She became less preoccupied with how she appeared to her own inspecting gaze and to onlookers and those she wished would look upon her.

In 1792, feminist writer Mary Wollstonecraft described this invisible confinement of feeling that we're defined by our bodies at the expense of our humanity: "Taught from their infancy that beauty is woman's scepter, the mind shapes itself to the body, and roaming round its gilt cage, only seeks to adorn its prison." When our body images and self-images are defined primarily by how we look, our bodies become our prisons. Adorning them—through makeup, fashion, cosmetic procedures, dieting regimens—becomes our full-time job and greatest work in the hopeful pursuit of love, confidence, and fulfillment. And as you do the work of constantly decorating and "improving" yourself, you are rewarded. You are validated by friends and strangers alike who see your looks changing and shout your praises — "You look amazing!" "I'm so jealous!" "You've never looked better!" "Keep it up!" You are validated by the heads you turn and the second glances, the more-interested romantic partners, the new likes and follows, the people looking to you as an expert and asking you about your secrets to success.

But this validation is fleeting, and it can take you only so far. When your weight loss slows down or the Botox wears off, so do the compliments. When you think harder about the praise you have received, you wonder whether these people value you only for your looks, and whether they felt bad for you before. You realize you have to work even harder to continue to earn the validation that had been your motivating force. As you hit your goals — the weight loss, hair removal and treatments, breast enhancements, lip filler, new outfit you finally saved up to buy — you begin to grasp the hard truth: These things don't make you any happier in the long term. They don't earn you love. Even if they earn you more attention from romantic prospects, they don't guarantee you can keep it or be fulfilled by it. They don't free you from body shame. They cost you an incredible amount of money, time, and energy. Chasing beauty ideals in the hopes of ridding yourself of shame or becoming happier or more confident is exhausting and never actually solves your problems in the long run. The truth is, being defined by our appearance is the real problem, and the endless beauty work we do to improve our confidence and body image is just a symptom of the problem, not the solution.

Selfie-Objectification

Understanding the reality of self-objectification in your own life can really complicate what empowerment and validation look like. Let's take posting pictures of ourselves online as an example to bring this home. Many girls and women post photos of themselves online to chase that high that comes from fire emojis, #goals comments, likes, and follows. It can feel body image boosting and empowering to share our own bodies and faces online, whether they look like the conventional ideals or not. If women *not* feeling beautiful were the *problem* and if women feeling beautiful were the *solution* to our body image woes, sharing pics of yourself on social media would definitely create and constitute progress. But if you understand the consequences of self-objectification in your life, it's not that simple. Keep in mind that we all post photos of ourselves for more than just looks-based validation. We want to document and keep people updated on what we're doing, where we're going, who we're with, and so on. However, it's still important to consider how you curate your photos, and whether you are doing so in hopes of boosting your body image and confidence about your looks.

Consider this: What if the very act of snapping and sharing photos of yourself in an effort to boost your self-esteem is just a visual and virtual extension of the self-objectification so many of us live with regularly in our minds? What if you are just turning your mental image of your body into a visible image, monitoring and evaluating it and seeking personal and social validation for how it appears? If body image were something that could be viewed and understood from the outside, then we could improve it from the outside too. Validation from ourselves and others for how we appear would solve all body image issues, and we'd all move on with our lives without a care in the world about whether we look like the current ideals. But body image is an inside issue, and no outside praise for how our bodies appear will ever provide long-lasting confidence and fulfillment.

One of Dove's marketing videos, aptly named "Selfie," asks girls and women to "redefine beauty" by taking selfies and realizing how beautiful they are. One of the takeaway messages at the end of the video is from a girl saying, "I was looking through my selfies last night and I realized I am beautiful. I'm pretty cute." That's nice! It really is. But looking through your selfies and evaluating your beauty to remind yourself of your value is the perfect illustration for describing the harmful state of self-objectification.

The rise of selfies might even correlate with the rise in cosmetic surgery for young women. According to a 2018 report by the American Academy of Facial Plastic and Reconstructive Surgery (AAFPRS), cosmetic procedures have increased by 47 percent since 2013. Of the facial plastic surgeons surveyed, 72 percent said that they'd noticed an increase in patients under thirty years old. In a 2014 statement, Edward Farrior, president of the AAFPRS, said, "Social platforms, . . . which are solely image based, force patients to hold a microscope up to their own image and often look at it with a more self-critical eye than ever before.

These images are often the first impressions young people put out there to prospective friends, romantic interests and employers and our patients want to put their best face forward."

What is most frightening to us is the idea of putting "their best face forward," which really means "putting a *different* face forward" and "changing their faces to fit ideals they've been trained to perceive as the best." But let's be real, this is not about an individual's *best*— this is about the beauty industry's *best-selling* ideals. This is a dangerous, expensive, painful, and ultimately *ineffective* way to reduce body shame or keep your body image afloat.

Selfies aren't inherently wrong. Not at all. And taking fifty-five pictures of your own face at slightly different angles and with varying expressions is not fundamentally bad. But (you knew a "but" was coming) when we put this phenomenon in the context of the culture in which we live, selfies aren't just a trivial trend or a form of self-expression. Rather, they are a clear manifestation of exactly what we have been taught to be our entire lives: images to be looked at. Carefully posed, styled, and edited images of otherwise dynamic human beings for others to gaze upon, evaluate, and like or comment on. They're not just images you take of yourself for yourself to see; they are images you take of yourself for others to see. Artists' self-portraits excluded, selfies weren't a thing until social media made it possible to be looked at and receive validation in an easy, public way online. And what have girls and women been taught from day one brings them the most value? Looking good. Not being smart or funny or kind or talented—mostly just looking hot. Thus the validation we have been taught to seek is the approval of others regarding our appearance. Social media simply allows us to replicate and magnify this phenomenon through a visual, public medium. We call it selfie-objectification.

> **Selfie-objectification** (noun): the process of presenting oneself as an object for viewing through a selfie that is shared with others online, which manifests itself in three steps:
> 1. capturing photos of yourself to admire and scrutinize;
> 2. ranking and editing those photos to generate an acceptable final image; and
> 3. sharing those photos online for others to admire and validate.

If you take a lot of photos of yourself (or have an "Instagram husband" or other partner take them), do you see yourself in these three stages, detailed below?

Stage 1: Capturing and Scrutinizing

Selfies are a unique phenomenon because they work as a more permanent form of a mirror. The images that are captured don't just disappear in a glance — they fill phone memories, computer albums, and social media feeds. They aren't captured and forgotten; they are captured and analyzed over and over again by the photographer herself, who's looking at her face and body and imagining how other people perceive her. With selfies providing a way for people to scrutinize and evaluate their own faces at any given moment, as well as more opportunities to compare their looks to all the other female forms that fill our social media feeds, it's no surprise to us that one of the ways many women cope with this shame is through "fixing" their faces and bodies with cosmetic surgery.

Stage 2: Ranking, Editing, and Selecting a Winner

After our selfie taker has examined and evaluated her photos, she selects the perfect shot for public viewing. If she's like the majority of social media users, she'll edit her image before posting. One survey showed 70 percent of millennial women respondents edited their own photos to "enhance their looks" by making alterations like removing blemishes, changing skin tones or color, or making themselves look thinner in some places and curvier in others. And if she doesn't alter her photo, she is likely to choose the one with the most flattering angle, light, and pose, which is its own form of editing. We almost never get to see female reality in mainstream media, and those unreal ideals result in the pressure we feel to alter our images to look more like the normalized cartoonish "perfection" we see everywhere else, subsequently perpetuating the unreality on social media.

Stage 3: Sharing and Monitoring

After posting the winning shot, the selfie taker is likely to carefully monitor the likes and comments it receives and compare those tiny symbols of validation to those on others' photos. The more likes and the nicer the comments, the better she feels about herself, or rather, her appearance. But what happens when the number of likes isn't to her liking? Or the comments are critical, or there are no comments? What happens to her self-worth then? When that self-worth is largely based on others' perceptions of her appearance, and others don't seem to be appreciating it as hoped, her entire self-worth suffers.

Here's the bottom line: self-objectification is a serious threat to your ability to see more in yourself—who you really are and what you're really capable of as a human, not as a body to be admired. Selfies, as a product of our appearance-obsessed culture, are one more tool we use to self-objectify. You may not even realize it because of how normal and prevalent the phenomenon has become. It is further complicated by the fact that no one (us included) wants to shame anyone for appreciating their appearance or to make anyone feel as though they should hide or hold back. However, if we're serious about self-worth and positive body image (which we very much are), then we all have a responsibility to critically consider the ways we view and represent ourselves and the ways self-objectification might play into that.

The Cut of Self-Comparison

While we're being dragged down by monitoring our own appearance and hoping others see us the way we want to be seen, we are also inevitably comparing ourselves to others. Each instance of self-comparison makes a little cut in our body image life rafts, causing them to deflate. You scroll 153 weeks deep into your ex-boyfriend's new girlfriend's Instagram posts. *Cut. Ssshhhhhh.* (That's the sound of air deflating from your body image life raft.) You watch your cousin play with the kids at the pool and wish you could wear that swimsuit and look like that. *Cut.* You flip through the group photos you took with friends last weekend and size yourself up against the whole crew, wishing you had posed or dressed differently. *Cut.*

Beauty isn't a limited resource in our world. Neither is love, attraction, validation, peace, intelligence, or happiness. But a world with narrow and highly prized ideals about bodies divides us into hierarchies of who looks right and who doesn't, and then ties our hopes for achieving all of those good things to our ability to climb the hierarchy. This pits us against our own bodies and each other in a constant state of comparison—whether to our past selves, our future body goals, or the woman in the office down the hall. This limiting, demeaning, divisive way of being causes us to become the watcher and the watched, the seer and the seen. We watch ourselves and compare the person we see to everyone else around us.

Not so shockingly, the majority of social comparison research about girls and women up to now focuses primarily on how they compare their looks and bodies, because that is where much of the pain and shame women experience originates. It is no surprise that many body image researchers, us included, have found that comparing our bodies with other women's leads directly to deflating body image. A whole body of research over decades has found that women who compare themselves to others have greater body anxiety and body dissatisfaction. Research also tells us that the social comparisons women tend to make are considered "upward social comparisons"—that is, comparisons to peers we believe look like us or are more attractive than us. This comparison never ends well, resulting in increased feelings of competition and body shame.

A recent experimental study on body dissatisfaction and woman-vs.-woman competition explored this sizing up in an interesting way. In the study, women were randomly exposed to two female research assistants who were either dressed in a manner that accentuated their thin figures (in attire similar to what would be worn at a job interview) and wore makeup, or dressed in non-form-fitting track pants and wore no makeup. In each of these two conditions, an attractive male was either present or not. Women who were exposed to the dressed-up research assistants reported they experienced greater body dissatisfaction than those exposed to the "frumpy" research assistants. The results indicated that body dissatisfaction in that scenario stemmed directly from self-comparison. Comparing rates of body dissatisfaction across the experimental groups, the researchers also found that women in the experiment with the dressed-up research assistant *and* the attractive man were the least satisfied with their bodies.

When we self-compare, we self-objectify. We rank our internal image of ourselves against someone else's external image —often a highly curated and edited image. Some of this is natural and unavoidable, but much of it is crippling to our body image and overall well-being. It creates distance between knowing ourselves as active subjects and viewing ourselves as passive objects. It pushes our body image farther out to sea in the waters of objectification, farther from our embodied self-perceptions. So much of our self-comparison and feelings of competition with and isolation from other women stem from our own shame and insecurities.

The women in our research explained how these self-comparison cuts deflated them in heartbreaking ways:

"My high school's five-year reunion was supposed to be last summer. I wanted to be brave and go, but knew I probably wouldn't. If I had gone with my husband, I know I would have left feeling crappy about myself . . . When I would think of going to the reunion, I would think about seeing all of those girls who were always pretty in high school, knowing they would probably only be prettier now. I think I would have left feeling like I'm a disappointment to my husband, because he would have noticed them, and then maybe he would have wondered if he could have gotten someone better."

"I stay home from activities often. My latest example is about indoor rock climbing. I am a full-figured woman, they rarely have a harness in XL that goes over my hips and butt. I have to squeeze into a large and then I feel even worse because I fear that I look like a sausage coming out of cellophane wrap. I look around at the other climbers and out of the hundreds that show up there

are two or three big girls like me. After my second time, I stopped going and started making all kinds of excuses."

"My entire life I have compared myself to others and always singled out my flaws. My appearance is something I feel is constantly weighing on my mind and I hate to admit it but probably 95% of the time I feel fat and unattractive. I do have my moments where I feel at least 'pretty' but for the most part I'm very hard on myself."

"I'm displeased with my physical appearance, particularly with regard to my weight. I feel like I look disproportionate, flabby, chubby, and broad in comparison to most other women near my age. I still get embarrassed letting my husband see my body, and he is the most supportive, noncritical guy I know."

"From ages 17 to 20, I competed in scholarship pageants. The neat part was that I did win a few and received money for college. The pitfall was that self-objectification became my life. I constantly compared myself to women in media and the pageant. The comparisons became very harmful. I was so paranoid to eat even a piece of candy for fear that my swimsuit competition would be threatened. I didn't feel well, I wasn't happy, I didn't have a normal menstrual period for months, and I constantly told myself 'I'm not enough.' I wasn't diagnosed as anorexic, but it's scary to realize I was on that track."

But what if you come out on top in comparison to someone else? You'd think being ranked higher would be good for your self-esteem, but that is not the case. Even when we deem ourselves to be higher in the hierarchy than someone else, based on size, shape, age, skin color, hair texture or style, or any other visible variable, we still lose. We might feel like winners in the moment, but we're buying into our own oppression and silently picking up the same sharp measuring stick to be used against us. We become numb to seeing others as objects in the same way we see ourselves. We subject ourselves and others to the same scrutiny we have been subjected to, and ultimately it hurts us all.

Research shows that women not only feel worse about their bodies after comparing them to others', but also feel less connection and unity toward the women they're measuring themselves against. ***If everyone is a competitor, no one is really on your team.*** When you harshly judge yourself, your self-consciousness is magnified, and this preoccupation with your looks leads you to feel isolated and competitive. The very act of self-comparison, even when it's a favorable comparison, not only causes our body image to plummet, but it also causes us to feel divided, alone, antagonistic, and distanced from other women — both in real life and online.

The increasing time we spend on heavily visual social media isn't helping. The American Academy of Pediatrics has referred to the major incidences of depression and body dissatisfaction faced by girls and women as "Facebook Depression," though it's absolutely not limited to Facebook. Studies show the more time users spend on social media, the more likely they are to experience decreased self-esteem, which is inevitable in the face of highly stylized, edited highlight reels being available to us twenty-four hours per day. Girls and women are likely to spend much more time on social media than boys and men, and to focus on the attractiveness of those in the photographs (while boys and men focus on career information that might deem the person "successful"). One study on young adults' relationships between self-esteem and Instagram use found that people who based their self-worth more on others' approval tended to self-compare on Instagram, which led to lower self-esteem. Other recent research has found that people who use social media more often tend to self-compare and self-objectify more often, too, which leads to worse mental health, lower self-esteem, greater body shame, and a greater likelihood of undergoing cosmetic surgery.

We want people to feel good about themselves, including about their appearance. But what we *really* want people to know is: Regardless of how you look, or how you *think* you look, you can feel good about yourself because *you are not your appearance.* **Your beauty is not your life's work.** You don't have to be beautiful. As blogger Erin McKean wrote at her site, A Dress a Day, "Prettiness is not a rent you pay for occupying a space marked 'female.'" As you begin to see the way your identity has been split in two—the viewer and the viewed—you can start to see yourself and experience your life in a new way. Once you see what self-objectification is and how it has impacted your life, you can't unsee it. Seeing it allows you to see more in yourself. It allows you to see the ideals and pressures causing you to *look* at yourself at the expense of *being* yourself. It's the being that makes you feel alive, that reminds you who you are and why you are here, and it's hard to be when part of you is always stuck surveilling your appearance.

Be More You

> We stop waiting to become as soon as we realize we already are.
> —Sonya Renee Taylor, *The Body Is Not an Apology*

When your identity is divided through self-objectification, you lose yourself. While you are eyeing your body up and down and narrowing in on certain parts, like the cameras do to women's bodies on your favorite trashy reality TV shows, you forget you even inhabit your body. When your view of yourself is limited or obscured by your external view of your looks, it can be hard to feel connected to yourself, your purpose, and life possibilities, let alone your body. Feeling defined by your appearance limits your perception of who you are and what you are capable of accomplishing. It halts your ability to work toward self-actualization. In order to reunite with your whole, embodied self, you must reclaim and redefine your identity beyond your appearance. Who are you? How did you get to where you are today? What do you want for your future? What are your strengths, skills, values, goals, purposes, passions, missions, motivating forces?

We so often start out as little girls with big dreams—just as big as those of little boys—and then right around the time puberty starts and our bodies begin to change, we start to change our minds. We hold back a bit, not raising our hands in class in order to avoid having all eyes on us, quitting the volleyball team because we have to wear spandex bloomers when the boys' team gets full shorts, not going to that event because we don't know what to wear. This shrinking of our possibilities and potential often continues throughout our whole lives as we opt out of leadership opportunities, career possibilities, playing with our kids, and other arenas in which our confidence has been undermined by our fears of what other people think of our looks.

As adults, our imagined goals in life often include our goal bodies, and many of us can't envision our happiest, most fulfilled future selves without also imagining ourselves looking different ("better") from how we do now. It is easy to mistake your purpose in life as *looking great* rather than *being great*—or believe you can't or won't reach your greatest purpose or live your best life if you don't also reach your hottest self. You can be anything you want! Girl power! *But you better look good doing it, or it doesn't count.*

It is undeniably hard to see your purpose—your reasons for being—outside of your looks when the message you are repeatedly sold is the opposite. It's hard to be more of who you really are or who you can become when the ways you've been taught to show up in the world are all about beautifying it (or reminding you that you must be beautiful and desirable no matter what you are doing). When media has consistently shown you that successful, loved, happy women all fit the same prescribed set of beauty ideals, it's hard to imagine you can meet your goals without meeting your "body goals."

But if your mission in life is primarily to take up less space, beautify the background, or mold yourself into something you've been taught is worthy of love and acceptance, you will never be fulfilled. That bar is consistently and purposefully set out of reach for living, breathing, aging, growing humans, and can move at any time. In order to cut through the distractions, you need to truly understand that your purpose, passion, and potential are not elevated or diminished by how you look on the path to getting there. The beauty contest built into our shared imagination has no trophy at the end, and the panel of judges and the criteria by which they are judging us are subjective and change constantly.

Under these conditions, how can you break the constraints that are keeping you from being more of who you really are, inside and out, and experience all the power and potential within your reach? You can reconnect with yourself and your holistic identity using the skills of self-reflection and self-compassion and by healing and finding purpose in your pain and your life.

Escaping Self-Comparison with Self-Reflection

As you think about what your life could be like and who you want to be, watch out for the distraction of comparing yourself to everyone else, who are on their own paths. When you feel the little stab of self-comparison, use it as a reminder to stop for a moment and reevaluate. Rather than looking outward to measure your progress and status, you can look inward by practicing self-reflection. This method of inquiring within can help put your purpose and chosen path back within view, regardless of where anyone else is on their own path or how they appear in the process. It also strengthens your resilience by helping you see the capacities, traits, resources, and skills you already have as well as the ways you might be limited. This strategy can be used during or after a disruption to your body image, as you work to rise with resilience, or routinely, as part of ongoing efforts to be more mindful and to think critically.

By turning to conscious self-reflection rather than unconscious self-comparison, it is possible to figure out what is distracting you from your greater purpose and power and get yourself back on course—and it gets easier the more you practice. Look yourself right in the eye and carefully consider your choices, feelings, and beliefs. What does it feel like when you compare yourself to others? How does it feel when you measure yourself against a celebrity's or friend of a friend's Instagram while you are in a slump, lounging makeup-free in your sweats? Or when you look around at school, church, the pool, that fancy event, or the people your partner follows on social media and imagine where you fall in the beauty (or success or happiness or popularity) rankings? Or when you get invited to an event and start worrying about what you'll wear and how you'll do your hair because you know everyone else will look amazing?

It might be a sinking feeling in your gut that gets your mind racing about what others must be thinking of you, a twinge of jealousy that sparks a to-do list or shopping bender to improve your appearance, or a darkening feeling that convinces you to stay in tonight, cancel a date, or skip an activity tomorrow. When you feel it, stop. Stop scrolling, stop watching, stop measuring and evaluating and comparing. Recognize that you are splitting against yourself — judging and blaming your body for your fears of how you might not measure up.

Stop the split by taking time to consciously reflect on the ways you have coped with these disruptive feelings in the past. Your response to those sinking feelings might have been to keep sinking to the bottom with self-harm or substance abuse, or a cycle of bingeing and restricting food, or texting that old fling who doesn't treat you well, or other destructive behaviors to numb and distract yourself. Or you might have reacted by clinging to your comfort zone, making quick fixes — like teeth whitening, cleanses and restrictive diets, or chemical peels and pricey new skin regimens — to alleviate your anxiety, or hiding out by taking a pass on invitations out with friends, not starting that small business, opting out of that spin class you used to go to, or postponing that art class until you feel more confident again.

Reflecting in this way allows you to name and identify not only your disruptions, but also your potential alternative responses, which gives you the chance to consciously respond in a different way. When you develop the capacity to see your disruptions as opportunities for personal growth, you are becoming more powerful, present, and resilient.

You can learn to be self-reflective and increase your confidence in your reactions and abilities each time you experience a wave of disruption by practicing these four steps of self-reflection:

1. **CHECK IN WITH YOURSELF.** When you experience something painful or triggering or uncomfortable as it relates to your body or your body image, ask yourself the following questions: On an emotional level, what am I feeling right now? *(Am I angry? Sad? Motivated? Hopeful?)* Physically, how do I feel? *(Am I tense? Nauseous? Sweating? Is my heart rate elevated?)* How am I reacting and responding? What do I feel compelled to do?

2. **NAME THE WAVE.** Ask yourself, "What is the specific instance or situation that caused me to experience this wave of disruption to my body image?" *(What happened to cause me to feel this way? Who said it? Who or what triggered it? How was I feeling before this wave hit me? Am I in a particularly emotionally vulnerable place? What deeper fears or feelings is this disruption bringing to light?)* Instead of trying to pin a disruption on a broad situation like "being invited to go swimming" or a million other examples, you can learn to see how many factors combine to trigger you at different times and in different ways. Maybe "being invited to go swimming" is a trigger because of who is inviting you, who might see you, how self-conscious you felt last time you wore your swimsuit, the fact that your body has changed, how you may not have the right swimsuit, or those negative comments you

just saw on that Instagram post of that girl who looks like you. Take a moment to really consider what is pushing you under the water. As you look back on the wave that knocked you down, you can learn to redefine what it is, what it means to you, and how you can react to it.

3. **RETHINK YOUR REACTION.** When you've felt similar pain or shame in the past, how did you react? What were your go-to coping mechanisms for dealing with body image blows? As you consider how you have responded in the past, ask yourself a few important questions to help you determine how you can now move forward in a way that serves you. Ask yourself: When I've dealt with similar feelings of shame or pain in my past, why did I respond that way? Did my response serve me or hurt me? What could I do differently this time? How can I see this as an opportunity for growth? What did I learn from this experience and my reaction to it? Do I have the resources to respond to this disruption in a healthier way?

4. **CHART YOUR COURSE.** If you feel like your responses to past waves of disruption served you, take note of how you responded and why it worked so well, and use that as motivation to deal with the pain you feel now in a more powerful way. If you feel like your response caused you to sink or flounder, or didn't help you change in positive ways, think about how you might respond differently. This is your opportunity to choose a new path. Choosing a different response to a wave

of disruption might feel less comfortable than simply rolling with old tried-and-true behaviors. The ways you've learned to cope may not ultimately be helpful, but they call it a comfort zone for a reason, and each disruption is an opportunity to get out of that seemingly safe state and into a more fulfilled way of being.

Let's walk through a potential opportunity to self-reflect and choose a more resilient response to a body image disruption: Your mom just emailed you and your siblings about getting together to do family pictures. Your stomach sinks as a wave of body shame settles in, whispering to you that you're too gross to take family pictures in your current state. That wave of shame is your cue to stop everything and practice the four steps of self-reflection.

CHECK IN: *That feeling I'm feeling right now — that's shame. I feel embarrassed and stressed. I feel it in my stomach, this sinking feeling. I feel it in my shoulders tightening up and my jaw clenching. My heart rate is up. I'm tempted to start a crash diet and make a hair appointment, and maybe I should hurry up and get Botox now so it'll settle before we have to take the pictures.*
NAME THE WAVE: *I'm nervous about capturing my weight gain and aging face in pictures that everyone will frame and post online for the world to see. I'm embarrassed that I haven't been working out and dieting like I used to and people are going to notice. I'm ashamed to be standing next to my younger/thinner/prettier sister-in-law.*

But what do these things have in common? They reveal my belief that my body defines me. My fear that other people value my body above anything else about me and will assign labels to me based on how I look, like that I'm lazy or gave up on myself. These feelings reveal this imaginary obligation I feel to beautify myself for potential onlookers.

RETHINK YOUR REACTION: *I've felt this way before. Remember when I had to do that filmed presentation at that conference and I went on a two-week cleanse and spent way too much on a new outfit and stressed myself out so bad I couldn't sleep before the event? It turned out it was all fine, and I didn't need to get so worked up. I lost a little weight, but I gained it back, plus more. No one at the conference was as intimidating as I pictured them being in my head, and I could have gotten away with wearing any work outfit I already owned. And yeah, I didn't look like a perfect model on camera, but who cares? People were there to hear me—not see me. That opportunity boosted my confidence in my speaking ability and introduced me to new contacts I wouldn't have made otherwise. Maybe I need to look at this family picture ordeal in the same way. I need to reframe this photo as an opportunity to help me realize I have some underlying shame and fear I need to uproot. Who cares if I don't love the picture? Who cares if someone thinks I'm uglier/older/fatter than my sister-in-law? So what if I gained weight or look older? I did gain weight and I am older—I'm human! I'm lucky* *to have a family and to be alive and well enough to take a picture with them. My family loves me no matter what I look like, and vice versa. This picture isn't about me — it's about all of us together.*

CHART YOUR COURSE: *I'm going to show up for this. I can use this picture as a reminder of the truth I'm working to believe: I am more than a body. I'm going to do it without punishing myself into meeting some weight or beauty goal. I will not be held back by my worst fears of what someone else might think when they see me. I can use this opportunity to prove to myself and everyone else that I am not defined by my body, that my appearance is just one facet of my being, and that I am okay as I am. I'm not in competition with my family members, because they are more than bodies, too, and we are all navigating this objectifying world together. And showing up on camera with a genuine smile can give other people the courage to show up too. I'm excited to have a picture with my family and I want this photo to capture the contentment and love I feel.*

As you walk through the four steps of self-reflection, keeping your self-worth and all the great things you are capable of in mind, you will gain a better perspective and motivation to make positive changes to the ways you cope. If you need some ideas, we can suggest a few reasons why you can and should choose a healthier, more empowered response to the pain you experience.

1. Because you deserve to grow from pain and show yourself you can rise in the face of it!
2. Because nothing and no one should make you feel unworthy or devalued!
3. Because you have come this far and you are capable of even greater power and fulfillment!
4. Because the world needs you to show up and contribute good *despite* what you've been through!
5. Because the world needs you to show up and contribute good *because* of what you've been through!
6. Because you can be an example to those watching from the sidelines who can benefit from seeing you persevere!

(It helps to get really enthusiastic with yourself if you need the extra motivation.)

Beauty Work Inventory

As you reflect on the ways self-objectification impacts your life, it is important to consider all the ways you have bought into beauty expectations just to feel like "yourself" or present the best possible version of "you." You might have been doing the same kinds of beauty work your whole life, or maybe your time and efforts relating to beauty have escalated recently. It can be really difficult to be critical and conscious of our beauty choices while navigating a world where objectification is normalized and a certain level of beauty work is expected of most women. To be clear

—it is okay and normal to desire validation for how you present yourself to the world. We are not going to pretend like our bodies are invisible or that anything beauty-related should be shunned. Absolutely not. It is wonderful to have the freedom and ability to make these choices, and the kind of affirmation that comes from others who like the way we look can be really nice (when it is welcomed—not when it is yelled from a car or messaged from an aggressive stranger). But remember that none of our choices are made in a vacuum. We live in a world that prizes our bodies above our humanity, so the motives behind all of our appearance-related choices need to be critically viewed through that lens.

When it comes to grooming choices, it is up to each of us to figure out what is oppressive and what is creative self-expression or simply personal preference. When are you coping with shame by trying to hide or fix your "flaws"? When are you having fun using fashion and makeup as creative self-expression? Taking inventory of your beauty-related choices can help you reflect and draw a line for yourself to determine what might be oppressive and what is fun and worthwhile.

Consciously answer these questions in your own mind or in writing, with no one to answer to but yourself:

- Does the amount of time, money, and energy I'm investing in my beauty and diet regimens feel appropriate, burdensome, or somewhere in between?
- Could any of my valuable resources be invested in better ways?

- Which parts of my beauty routine and diet do I rely on to look or feel like "myself" or the best version of "myself"?
- Can I explore cutting any of them down or out of my life, just to see how it feels?
- Is there anything I especially enjoy or appreciate about my beauty routine?
- Where do I draw the line between what is creative and fun in my beauty work and what is driven by shame, self-consciousness, and wanting to live up to a hoped-for ideal?
- Am I happy with where that line is drawn, or could I consider setting a new boundary for my beauty work or diet?

As you go over your inventory, carefully look to see if it shows that you might be basing too much of your self-worth on what you or others think of your appearance, or that you are spending too much precious time, money, pain, or energy on beauty-related matters. This is subjective, and it is truly up to you to decide these things. Your answers might even change over time. If you don't like something you've found, or if you see possibilities to adjust your thinking, spending, or efforts, then you've got a great opportunity to make some conscious changes. When we truly know that we are more than bodies, we can carefully consider our body-related choices through that lens and take back some of our power in the process rather than unconsciously buy into beauty expectations.

This will absolutely require sacrifices and a willingness to be vulnerable. For example, it could be awkward and uncomfortable to scale back on your makeup and have people ask, "Are you feeling okay?" just because your face is less made-up than usual. If you are taking steps to opt out of traditional beauty work, you might need to let people know you're looking out for yourself right now by prioritizing how you feel over how you look and figuring out how to understand and value your body differently. Invite them to join you as you prove to yourself and the world around you that your beauty routine doesn't make you more "you."

As we evaluate our own choices around our appearance, we have to be careful to avoid shaming or blaming anyone for the choices they make in the name of beauty, validation, and their own representation online or in real life. We don't need to approve of each other's choices or police anyone else's personal beauty routines or personas. That's not helpful. What *is* helpful is having an open dialogue with ourselves and those under our care about our own individual choices and what influences them. These are important questions every woman must consider, and we have to do it in advance of increasing pressures with aging and beauty and body "innovations" becoming more commonplace and expected in some circles.

The Comfort of Self-Compassion

When you practice self-reflection, you may not like the honest answers you find. You might not be happy with the ways you've spent your time, money, and energy trying to fit a mold that doesn't fit you or serve you. You might not like how large a role

shame has in driving your habits and behaviors and how difficult it is to change them. Whether or not you like what you find
through self-reflection, you can make the choice to treat yourself
with compassion. Self-compassion means having your own back
—accepting yourself and your past choices unconditionally.
This way of being can help you survive disappointments, disruptions, less-than-ideal responses to those disruptions, and deflated
comfort-zone life rafts. It won't prevent the difficulties that we all
face, but it can help you get through them.

Self-compassion helps you develop and access body image
resilience by reminding you to be patient, understanding, and
loving with yourself, regardless of the circumstance or what
brought you there. The sense of security and relief it can bring
is life changing. Research pioneered by Dr. Kristin Neff shows
that developing and accessing self-compassion can help counter
destructive self-critical tendencies, including self-comparison.
Have you ever been burdened and overwhelmed by a situation or
problem, only to be comforted by someone else's simple acknowledgment that what you're going through is hard? That response
is validating and affirming, and you can do that for yourself too.

Rather than berating yourself for feeling a certain way or act-
ing on your feelings in a way that doesn't serve you, try taking a
deep, compassionate breath. Speak kindly to yourself, acknowledge the reality of the pain you feel and the unfairness of objectification, and validate your past and present responses to that
pain: *This is hard, and I hate feeling this way. What I am experiencing is
unfair, but I am okay. I am doing my best. I can always improve how I react*

to the difficulties of my life, but I am alive. I am breathing. I have come this far. I am not alone.

Neff writes, "Self-compassion means being more willing to experience difficult feelings and to acknowledge them as valid and important. The beauty of self-compassion is that instead of trying to get rid of 'bad' feelings and replacing them with 'good' ones, positive emotions are generated by embracing our suffering with tenderness and care, so that light and dark are experienced simultaneously." **We can change and grow and react differently because we respect and care for ourselves — not because we hate who we are and are trying to punish ourselves.**

When you catch yourself in a state of self-objectification or self-comparison, or when you don't like the answers revealed in your self-reflection, acknowledge what you are experiencing and respond to yourself with self-compassion in whatever way works best for you. Find a mantra or phrase that resonates with you. Listening to or reading positive affirmations can help you discover the kind of inspiring messages that speak to your heart.

Try listening to guided meditations (even passively, while you are doing other things) from people like Belleruth Naparstek, whose affirmations, meditations, and guided imagery are healing and calming. Certain phrases will jump out and strike you. By writing them down and rereading them, you can turn to those phrases to aid in your own self-compassion. When you feel that sinking feeling of your identity being split into the seer and the seen, the you and the you that is being looked at, use self-compassion to talk yourself back into your body. Even just engaging in a casual, caring dialogue with yourself can be helpful. Try something like, *Wait—I can feel that I'm picturing myself being looked at instead of just living. It's so easy to do, but I deserve more than this. It does not matter how I look right now. I deserve to look out and see the sky, the people walking past, and feel the air on my skin. I deserve to breathe for a moment and think about other aspects of my life.*

When you are dealing with body anxiety, you might find that you are lost in thought, hypothesizing about worst-case scenarios, and worrying about abstract fears, not dealing in concrete reality. In those cases, you can work to immediately let go of unnecessary anxieties by getting out of the clouds and into your own senses. If you're walking somewhere, look at everything you're passing on the street. Look at people rather than imagining how you look through their eyes. Watch cars pass by and look inside the storefront windows. Smell the air, feel your hands in your pockets or swinging by your sides. Pay attention to the rhythm of your feet hitting the ground with each step. Turn your thoughts toward what you are experiencing physically and remind yourself how grateful you are to be free from pain (when you are), to be able to walk (or modify this example if you cannot), and to have comfortable clothes and shoes. Make sure your self-dialogue is kind and understanding.

If you are trying on jeans at a store or from the back of your closet and you are dismayed to find that the size you usually wear doesn't fit or is squeezing your thighs or waist in a way you feel ashamed of or that your curves can't fill them out in the ways you want, remind yourself that you are privileging an onlooker's perspective of your body. Repeat to yourself that you are more than a body, and you are, in fact, human. A human who reserves the right to have a body that grows and shrinks and changes. A person who will not be dismayed by the consistently inconsistent sizes between one brand of clothing and the next. A person who cannot be defined or confined by jeans that don't fit right. A person who deserves to be comfortable in whatever size pants is the best fit.

Then tap into your senses to step back into your body as your own. Turn away from the mirror to help you reunite with your body as an insider instead of being an outsider looking in. Close your eyes and breathe. Stretch your hamstrings, your calves, your glutes. Feel the stretch. If you are able, do a lunge and feel the power of your muscles at work. Consider where your legs have taken you lately and express gratitude to them for the work they do. Reflect on memories of fun hikes or bike rides or park outings you've been on, and on the privilege of having legs to get you where you need to go. Do anything you can to place yourself and your consciousness back inside your body.

If you are having an intimate moment with a romantic partner and you feel yourself slip away as a distant observer, anxious and hyperaware of what your partner must be thinking about your body, take back your presence and pleasure. Give yourself a little mental pep talk: You deserve to enjoy this moment. Your sexuality cannot be observed from the outside. It's not something you are worthy of experiencing only if you feel like you fit some manufactured standard of what "sexy" looks like. Your sexuality is your own, and you can reconnect with it by reconnecting with your own body. Step back into *your* senses rather than trying to guess what your partner is thinking or feeling or seeing. How do you feel? If you feel good, communicate it to your partner. If they could do something differently to help you feel more comfortable or connected, communicate it. Ask for them to do the same and listen to them. Your partner is choosing to be with you in this moment, so each time you feel their hand on a part of you that you feel self-conscious about or find yourself worrying about what they must be seeing from that angle, reclaim this experience as yours, too. You aren't performing for them; you are in this together. You deserve to feel pleasure and live in the moment, because the moment is yours, too.

Reaching Out

Choosing to be kind to yourself can also give you space to look around and recognize that you are truly not alone and to ask for help when you need it. Your experiences in the waters of objectification are not that unique. We all feel so singularly affected by shame and anxiety so much of the time, but we are not in any way exceptional in this. You are the norm! Even in your darkest moments, many people have been where you are. Despite this, it takes a lot for any of us to admit to struggling. We fear being judged, looked down upon, and being told our feelings are dumb or wrong or unnecessary. So we put on a show of being cool, confident, and carefree as long as we possibly can. It's hard to tell the truth and reveal that you aren't perfect or that you are fearful about how others see you and the repercussions of not living up to the ideals. Practicing self-reflection and self-compassion can help you see the deeply ingrained feelings of embarrassment and fear that stay buried deep in your consciousness and wreak havoc on your self-perception. And when you can reflect on the painful experiences that are casting a shadow over your current beliefs and actions relating to your body, you might also see a need to turn that reflection outward to catch someone else's attention.

Not all of your burdens can or should be carried alone. The industries built around body shame rely on all of us feeling abnormal (as if "normal" is what we're really comparing ourselves to) and embarrassed about not living up to the ideals—so much so that we keep it inside and pretend to be confident and happy even when we're drowning. So many of us feel compelled to suffer alone out of shame, but our silence holds shame in power. When dark feelings arise from self-comparison or even from self-reflection, you can use them as an opportunity to open up to trusted people—online, in real life, through a call or a letter or a text, or even in an anonymous discussion forum. Signal to others that you could use some help or solidarity.

When a participant in our research opened up about serious pain caused by her parents' constant attention to her weight and criticism of her body, we encouraged her to be open with her family about what she was experiencing. A few weeks later, she wrote back, saying, "I just wanted to let you know that two nights ago I had a really good talk with my parents. We were able to be really open and honest about body image, and it's helped both of us forgive past hurts. It's still a process, but I can tell this is a really good step. I wanted to thank you again, because I wouldn't have talked to them if I hadn't written out the feelings and experiences you told me to write. I told them about my experience with this study and we're all ready to move on and forward!"

By honestly unloading her real, raw feelings about her body image and the ways her parents had created and exacerbated that pain, she prompted them to make positive changes to benefit the whole family. Whether it is to a family member, romantic partner, good friend, or other trusted individual, opening up about our darkest thoughts and experiences can help take the sting out of them. If the hurt and pressure are being caused by someone close to us, being honest about our body image struggles can open the door to change and give them the opportunity to acknowledge the burden or even help us carry it.

Unfortunately, not everyone you open up to or signal to for help will be willing or able to assist you. They might not have developed their own ability to be self-compassionate or discerning about body ideals, and that can prevent them from being equipped to help you or anyone else, even if they want to. They might be resistant to any challenge to their own assumptions and ideas about body image. It's okay. Not everyone can help, but hearing about your sincere struggle might plant a seed in their mind that grows over time into a desire to gain more knowledge and understanding. Don't let others' hesitancy or inability to help stop you from finding the people who will.

Sometimes you need assistance not only from the people you love, but also from professionals who can provide greater support. For example, eating disorder recovery is often not possible alone, regardless of how many resources and supporters you have around you. Overexertion can be addictive and a slippery slope from regular, moderate exercise for those who are susceptible to it in response to shame or anxiety. Self-harm might be too powerful of a draw in hard moments, no matter how aware you are of its danger or its inability to provide lasting comfort or escape. Substance abuse disorders and addictions of all kinds, including to prescription drugs, illegal drugs, and alcohol, can take down even the strongest and smartest of people. And even people who don't face immediate, visible challenges can often benefit from professional support. We all have complicated emotions and cope with pain in ways that don't serve us. Therapy is for everyone.

One of our study participants specifically acknowledged the power of having a therapist teach her careful self-reflection and how greatly it impacted her success in recovering from a decade-long eating disorder and distorted self-image. She said, "I was trained to be very in tune with my emotions—when I was feeling them, why I was feeling them, how to manage what I was feeling. I am very grateful that I was given opportunities to develop this skill and sharpen my emotional intelligence. It has been a great blessing in my life."

Don't let any lingering stigma against therapy or inpatient or outpatient treatment for addiction or disordered eating hold you back from finding relief and freedom through professional support. Hard-fought and hard-won miracles transpire in people's lives when they have finally pursued the treatment and therapy they needed. With the right professionals (and sometimes it takes a few tries), huge transformations can be possible. But getting that help requires you to signal for it, whether by talking to others about treatment options and getting recommendations for good providers, or even by checking yourself into the hospital. Point that reflector toward someone you trust, catch their attention, open up with as much honesty and vulnerability as you can, and keep doing that until you find the right help to manage your burdens and find relief.

In a piece for NBC News, superstar musician Lizzo opened up about the complexities of self-compassion and acknowledging when you need help to feel that love.

I don't think that loving yourself is a choice. I think that it's a decision that has to be made for survival; it was in my case. Loving myself was the result of answering two things: Do you want to live? 'Cause this is who you're gonna be for the rest of your life. Or are you gonna just have a life of emptiness, self-hatred, and self-loathing? And I chose to live, so I had to accept myself . . . I want people first to understand that there are levels to loving yourself. To an extent, choosing not to hate yourself can be a choice, but, at a certain point, people can develop mental health issues from self-hatred, from bulimia or anorexia to depression. Sometimes, you need therapy to help you learn to love yourself. I know that therapy is some privileged sh**, and the fact that I'm financially able to afford it, and that I was also in a place where I could accept the fact that I needed it, is incredibly fortunate . . . Self-care is really rooted in self-preservation, just like self-love is rooted in honesty. We have to start being more honest with what we need, and what we deserve, and start serving that to ourselves.

Reconnecting

Lizzo is right that "therapy is some privileged [stuff]," but even if traditional one-on-one psychotherapy isn't accessible, there are tools you can use on your own. Self-reflection and self-compassion can be incredible resources to help develop resilience, but we also need to look way beneath the surface in order to root out our faulty core beliefs about ourselves. One common, impactful therapeutic practice is called "inner child" work, which taps into the subconscious beliefs we have carried inside us since childhood. The basic psychological premise of this method is that the things we experienced and the messages we received as children play a role in our adult lives as well, and we often act out those beliefs in ways we don't recognize. If we can reconnect with our inner child to understand and address the things that impacted us negatively, we can heal and move forward without some of the constraints and burdens we have carried from childhood.

From Lindsay: This was something I learned about in college and read about over the years as others dealt with their own issues with relationships, food, anger, depression, and anxiety. I knew others found it helpful, and I recognized that experiences in my own childhood shaped my body image in negative ways and drew me into the waters of objectification. But even knowing this, I didn't directly confront my own "inner child" until I started therapy on my own. It melted. my. heart.

It wasn't even some deep line of questioning or intense process that led me to this melting. My wonderful therapist, Barbara, simply asked me to picture myself as a little girl, in a happy moment I can remember or in a photo I like. My mind immediately went to a picture of me as a five-year-old on Easter, sitting on a brown striped couch, smiling sweetly with a white bunny cradled in my arms. I am wearing baggy yellow pleated pants and a pink pastel sweatshirt zipped up to my chin. My blonde hair is pulled into a ponytail on top of my head and my bangs and some short side hair are curled and fluffed up (the '90s go-to look for little girls). I absolutely love this picture of me. I can't even believe it's me because I'm so little and adorable, yet it is so totally *me*. My dark eyebrows are starting to grow in thick and strong, my genuine smile pushes out my round cheeks, and I lovingly and carefully hold that little white bunny — an Easter present I cleverly named "Whitey" and whose siblings, "Blacky" and "Brownie" (guess their colors!), belonged to Lexie and our little brother, Garrett.

Barbara referred to this image of me as "your little girl" and said to imagine myself with my arm around my little girl, sitting next to her on that brown couch from my childhood living room. I was instantly in tears. I was then — and still am now — overwhelmed with unconditional love for "my little girl." Even just thinking of that name for her melts me all over again. She looks like Lexie's little daughters, whom I love so much, and thinking of myself in the same way I think about them opened my heart in a new way.

Barbara then asked me to think about the earliest time I can recall when my little girl felt embarrassed about something and to describe those feelings. When I explained fragments of memories and circumstances of when I felt ashamed in response to comments about my body or my food choices before adolescence, she said, "What would you say to your little girl about those moments? What do you want her to know that no one told you?" I wanted for my little girl what we all (hopefully) want for our little girls—to feel unconditionally safe, accepted, loved, validated, and understood. Saying it aloud in the words I might use for her was transformative.

Going home and writing "my little girl" a letter was even more transformative. I wrote:

Dear Little Lindsay,

I'm so sorry you feel embarrassed. The people who made you feel that way didn't know they were wrong to say those things and act that way, but they were. They learned that fat was a bad thing to be and they saw that you were a little bit fat. They didn't mean to hurt you, but you did get hurt. When you felt hurt, you learned to think about yourself and your body differently. You started to worry more about how you look and what other people think rather than just living your life like before.

But you are OK. You always were and you always will

be. No matter how you look or what you eat or how fast you can run or what anyone says. There is nothing wrong with you. You aren't broken or weak or embarrassing. Of course you want to eat the foods you learned were off-limits. Of course you feel ashamed of how you look when people around you want to be smaller.

But you deserve to feel comfortable in your own body. I trust you. You deserve to trust yourself. I want to help you learn what is true about you and what is not true. I want to help you learn to listen to yourself and understand your body from the inside, not from the outside. You are OK. No matter what. I love you. No one is embarrassed of you or for you. But even if they are, they are wrong—they learned wrong. They learned lies about bodies when they were little too. I'm excited to help you learn to feel happy about your body and for you to experience a really great life inside your body. That same body is going to be your home for your whole life. Isn't that amazing? It is yours. Your body is wonderful and good, but it isn't everything. You are everything.

Try it for yourself. Don't make it polished or rehearsed or perfect, just freewrite what comes to your mind and heart. Go through the details of your first experiences in the waters of objectification and how they made you feel. How did those first experiences shape the way you felt about and treated your body in the following years? How did you adapt and respond to your new awareness of others' judgments or the pressures of being consumed as an object? What do you want your "little girl" to know about herself and the coming waves of disruption in her life? What would you tell her about her worth, her power, her spirit, and her body? Speak it, write it, reread it, and believe it. That little, perfect, lovable person you're imagining is still you. The same you. Older, bigger, wiser, yes. But absolutely *you*, and exactly as worthy of love now as you were then.

A Spiritual Sense of Self

Seeking to more deeply connect with yourself might lead you not only to look beyond your immediate physical self, but also to explore your identity and purpose in a spiritual or metaphysical context—your reasons for existing, the meaning in your life and your pain, your higher self, and the power that exists beyond yourself. Though everyone might reach entirely different conclusions through entirely different beliefs and practices, the simple act of exploring a sense of self beyond the physical can provide comfort and greater perspective to many people. Objectification reduces people to the physical—the observable. Spirituality can counter that force with an emphasis on the parts of ourselves that are invisible but connected to greater meaning and power. It is connected to religion for lots of people, but it doesn't need to be associated with any organized practices or worship. The spirituality we are talking about simply refers to qualities concerning the human spirit or soul as opposed to material or physical things.

Spirituality can work as a buffer against all the appearance-focused messages we receive by expanding our sense of self, helping us feel valued and valuable for more than our physical bodies or how they appear. Laura Choate, author of *Swimming Upstream,* described this well, writing, "If a woman draws her sense of meaning from a spiritual force that goes beyond herself, and provides coherence and purpose to the universe, she will find less need to focus on her weight, shape, and appearance in an attempt to find happiness and life satisfaction."

For people whose spirituality is intertwined with religious practices and worship, their understanding of the nature of souls and their connection to a higher power might be shaped by their denomination, religious leaders, religious experiences, or scripture. For others, spirituality isn't necessarily connecting to God or a higher power, but instead is about tapping into their own "higher self" or innate divinity. It can be strengthening to imagine a more advanced or divine being—regardless of its form or identity—who is omniscient, kind, loving, and aware of you and your desires and needs, and with whom you can connect to gain balance, peace, and guidance. Others might feel connected to a source of energy in the universe, like the moon, the earth, or Mother Nature, or to another interconnected network of power from which they can access peace, healing, balance, or strength.

Regardless of how you conceptualize the spiritual in your life or how you choose to connect to a sense of self beyond your body, tapping into spirituality can be a powerful resource for developing resilience. When you can feel on a deep level that your reason for living isn't to be decorative, but that your existence has meaning, life opens up. Spirituality and faith repeatedly appeared in our research as traits that buffer against the damaging effects of objectification. Many women found comfort after being hit with waves of disruption when they turned to spiritual means for regaining a sense of balance and purpose in their lives. Whether through prayer, meditation, worship, scripture, healing blessings, yoga, tarot, or any other practice that reconnects you to an expanded sense of self or greater perspective, connecting to spirituality is a powerful way to find meaning in your pain and purpose in your life.

When you feel a bit of spiritual insight, inspiration, peace, or guidance, we encourage you to write it down or record it. Those moments that resonate with your innermost feelings are meaningful, and you can deepen their positive influence by keeping and remembering them. You can hone your skills for recognizing and utilizing spiritual power in your life by honoring the words, feelings, and experiences that pierce your heart and cut through the noise of body fixation. If it feels appropriate to share those experiences with others you trust, do it. Articulating the experiences that expand our views of ourselves can lend them greater power to aid in our process of developing resilience for future challenges.

From Lexie: In the spirit of honoring my own moments of inspiration, I want to share an experience I had when my first daughter was a baby. The experience was incredibly personal, but it was transformative for me and I hope it can help you as well. My husband, daughter, and I had spent a fun summer day at a lake. As we drove home with our baby girl in the back seat, I scrolled through the pictures my photographer husband had taken of us on his camera. I saw myself having fun in my swimsuit with my little girl. However, I was immediately caught off guard by the feelings of embarrassment that washed over me about how I looked, and with tunnel vision that obscured everything I believe in and stand for about my body and my worth, I quickly deleted all the photos I hated.

When we got home, I lay on my bed alone while my husband showered. I felt so overwhelmed by how ashamed I felt about how I looked, while also being ashamed that I was ashamed, and embarrassed that I deleted all of those photos without telling him. I knew it was out of character, and the shame was hitting me harder than I could have ever anticipated. As I was trying to get my bearings, I tried to tap into the greater understanding I have about my body and myself, even though it felt out of reach in this disruption. I half-talked/half-prayed aloud and felt this divine feminine feeling of comfort and love.

I asked for comfort, and as soon as I asked, the warmest feeling of love and pride washed over me. I then saw a mental image of myself walking somewhere — I was looking at myself from behind, as if I were outside my body, but in a state of loving awareness as opposed to self-objectification. As I looked at myself, I felt the same kind of pride I feel about my baby girl. I love every inch of her — her round belly, her soft legs, the fuzzy hair on the back of her head. I felt that for myself. As I watched myself walk, I felt this incredible warmth for who I was and what I was doing. I can describe it only as absolute, unconditional pride and love.

I laid there and cried tears of joy. My shame washed away. I felt pure love, and that love — love that I can only compare to the love I felt and still feel for my baby, which doesn't do it justice — is something I believe we can all ask for when we need it, from whatever source aligns with our beliefs. We all bear the burden of so much pain inside our bodies — pain inflicted physically, mentally, and emotionally — but we can tap into power beyond our own to expand our sense of self and access greater feelings of compassion and unconditional love for ourselves and, in turn, everyone else.

Please don't underestimate the power you have to make a difference in the world for those who need it. Many people are praying, mourning, feeling deflated, hoping, or seeking allies and helpers to lift them up and serve them in ways they need. You can be that person. Think about and practice accessing and expanding your sense of spiritual grounding, or other sources of purpose and meaning, to help shift the focus from yourself as a lone physical being and instead to our interconnectedness as part of a broader community. By improving your own sense of self, you can be better equipped to step outside your self-consciousness and reach out to others who need help.

In your life, how have you felt connected to the spiritual as opposed to the visual and physical sides of yourself and the world? How did it feel? How can you make space in your life for the practices that can help you reconnect with that side of yourself? One easy means for gaining that balance and knowing yourself better is through simply sitting with yourself and your thoughts. It is so easy to listen to and read other people's words all day long, filling the silence with music, podcasts, TV, and talking. But it is in silence that we often hear what we need to hear and feel what we need to feel from our own bodies and minds. In silence, it is much more difficult to distract ourselves from dealing with our disruptions and uncomfortable feelings and thoughts, but if we push them off for too long, they build up to a bigger wave that can do some real damage. So it's important to tune in and listen.

We all tune in differently, but some of the most common and effective ways to do that are through meditation, prayer, tai chi, journaling, yoga, spending time in nature, discussing spirituality and spiritual experiences with others, and entering a "flow" state through a peaceful activity. When you figure out what works for you, build it into your daily or weekly life in manageable ways and see how it helps you feel more grounded in your body and sense of self.

In that process, continue to exercise discernment and self-reflection. Dig deeply into your beliefs about yourself and the world. Assess your privileges and biases, engage in regular self-reflection, and continue to learn from reliable, diverse sources. All of this will help you get to the root of which beliefs and experiences have shaped you into who you are now.

Sometimes this digging will reveal what can be called the "shadow side" of something that is otherwise positive, like a belief or message that might have felt empowering or inspiring at one point or for one person but has a different effect for you later in life. In that vein, we offer a cautionary note: it is important to remain open as we examine the ways our own religious and spiritual practices have been shaped by cultural forces that might value some groups of people over others, instill harmful shame and guilt, enforce rigid gender roles that elevate men over women and define identities in limiting ways, or otherwise limit our beliefs about our own worth or potential or our views of other people's worth or potential. Churches, spiritual centers, religious leaders, gurus, and others who seek to guide and help others are not immune to the harmful influences that reinforce inequality, including the objectification of women and children.

If you feel your church or spiritual community perpetuates these harmful ideals, it is up to you to consider whether you can prompt some change from the inside, or whether it is best for you to find a new place of worship or spiritual home. Many people are in your same situation as they grow up and realize the comfort they once found at their church or in their spiritual study might also be complicated by teachings that are either no longer useful or outright harmful. Connecting with our communities and ourselves spiritually can be an incredible resource for resilience—just be sure it's also paired with discernment, reflection, and compassion for others who are different from you or don't share your beliefs.

Beyond the spiritual, there are countless ways to find purpose in your life to expand your sense of self and remind yourself of your power and potential. In what ways do you feel called to serve? What is important to you? How are you best equipped to do good in the world, to lead in ways that people need? What can you contribute that brings happiness, light, and peace to the world? Volunteer for a nonprofit whose mission resonates with you. Get involved in your community through the schools, local government, boards, activism, or helping kids or the elderly or a marginalized group. Find work or service that is meaningful and helps you do some good. Exercise your talents and create something — art, music, poetry, or creative writing. Your life is bigger than what you look like, and finding purpose is key to stepping outside the constraints of self-objectification.

All of these skills and tools — self-reflection, self-compassion, reconnection, and an expanded sense of self beyond the physical body — will help you get to know yourself better. To reunite with yourself in a way that helps you reclaim your body as your very own. To experience the privilege of your body, rather than privileging anyone else's view of you. You can *be more* of who you really are and who you always were.

You can know yourself and your power better by seeing and acknowledging your pain. You can take your own unique pain and use it to be *more* of who the world needs you to be — not less. **You can step into your power, capabilities, and purpose instead of hiding, fixing, or shrinking away.** What if your pain could point you toward your own personal path to gaining more compassion, more empathy, and more knowledge of your world, your capabilities, and yourself? You can use the very pain that was designed to hold you down to find purpose you could have never found otherwise.

Without so many years of body fixation, we personally would never have had our eyes opened to the harms of objectification and the reality of its effects on so many people's body- and self-perceptions. We wouldn't have learned how our identities had split at a very young age as we began to watch and evaluate our bodies from afar. We wouldn't have found the heart-pounding, life-giving drive to learn, teach, and advocate for others. We found missions and life-affirming purposes because of our body shame — not in spite of it — and for that, we are grateful for every moment of suffering that brought us to our present. That sense of purpose is what drives us to do the work we do. It pushes us beyond ourselves and our immediate fears, anxieties, and burdens to provide some guidance and solace to others who could use it.

As you seek and find your purpose (or many purposes), missions, reasons for being, and the paths that are often illuminated by your pain, you will be better equipped to be resilient in the face of body image disruptions. You will find yourself again and again. You will become less vulnerable to the stifling effects of self-objectification and self-comparison, and more confident in yourself as a whole, embodied person.

4

From Divided to United as Women

- Have you ever passed judgment on someone because
  of how they looked or dressed? Have you ever found out
  those judgments were wrong?
- Have you ever felt judged by someone because of how you
  looked or dressed?
- Write about both scenarios and describe how they felt. Did
  judging someone else's body or being judged by yours
  help you feel better or worse about other people and about
  yourself?

See More in Each Other

In our world, divide and conquer must become define and
empower.
—Audre Lorde, *Sister Outsider*

When we grow up in a world that teaches us our bodies are
the most important thing about us, it is easy to view other
people—even those we know and love—through that same ob-

jectifying lens we turn upon ourselves. *We feel defined by how we appear, and so we define everyone else, friend or foe, by how they appear, positively or negatively.* We tear people down by disparaging how they look, and we build them up by validating how they look. We become the oppressed and the oppressors; the victims of our objectifying culture and the perpetrators enforcing it upon each other. The insidious objectification of girls and women by *other* girls and women often looks like self-comparison and competition, questioning and commenting, policing and patrolling. It can also look positive and uplifting from the outside as we build each other up with compliments about how beautiful we are, but that sort of body commentary is still reinforcing the value of our appearance over all else. When we are so used to the constant, dragging burden of self-objectification and the nonstop waves and currents of our body-obsessed culture, we turn that limiting lens on the others in our lives—even those we love.

Imagine the collective weight we could lift off of each other's shoulders if we could learn to see more in everyone around us and treat them accordingly. We could have more genuine, fulfilling relationships as we bond over more than the way we appear. We could build new friendships and fulfill each other's needs better as we go beyond the surface. We could collectively strengthen each other against the objectifying messages that permeate our lives and reduce the ways we dehumanize each other by valuing bodies over all else. We could develop greater compassion and empathy for each other as allies instead of competitors. In this chapter, we will illuminate how objectification plays into the bullying and competition that divides us, the well-meaning body compliments that do more harm than good, how modesty and dress-code policing reinforce objectification, and how parent-child dynamics and romantic relationships can help or hurt body image.

Divided Against Each Other

Girls and women are often stereotyped as inherently catty, competitive, and vicious toward each other. Because of the environment that teaches us to see ourselves and others in limiting and objectifying ways, sometimes we inadvertently live up to those stereotypes by disparaging and cutting down other girls and women about their bodies. Sometimes we do this because we're unconsciously trying to bring someone down to our same deflated body image. After all, if we internalize the message that our looks and sexual appeal are the most important things we can offer the world, then the best way to cut someone else down is to attack her looks or sex appeal or the ways she uses both. Research shows that while men are more likely to be physically aggressive, women and girls are more likely to engage in indirect "relational aggression" (typically directed at other girls and women, especially those deemed attractive), which includes gossiping, criticizing each other's appearance, and alienating each other — a sex difference that shows up as early as age six.

In a review of several studies, researcher Tracy Vaillancourt summarized a variety of ways this manifests in everyday life: one study found that attractiveness increased adolescent girls' chances of being a target of indirect aggression by 35 percent, but decreased the odds by 25 percent for boys. It's similar for adults: one study from 2013 indicated that women in the workplace discriminated against same-sex job candidates, particularly those whom they deemed more attractive. Men, on the other hand, did not discriminate against men they deemed more attractive. And when it came to a request for forgiveness, women were less accepting of an apology and judged the apology to be less adequate when it was offered by a woman who was considered attractive than when it was offered by a supposedly "unattractive" woman.

Girls are more likely to be bullied than boys, according to statistics from the US Department of Education, and that bullying is most likely to happen online. Bullying has spread from school hallways and bathrooms to the virtual world, where a rise in cyberbullying across the US has resulted in three times as many girls than boys reporting being harassed by text message or online. According to the National Center for Education Statistics, 21 percent of girls in middle and high school reported being bullied online or by text message in the 2016–17 school year, compared with less than 7 percent of boys. And the reasons for being bullied reported most often by students included physical appearance at the top of the list. In particular, national surveys have found among overweight middle-school aged children that 30 percent of girls and 24 percent of boys experienced daily bullying, teasing, and/or rejection because of their size. These numbers doubled for overweight high school students, with 63 percent of girls and 58 percent of boys experiencing some form of bullying due to their weight and size.

The girl-on-girl bullying that takes place at depressing rates happens regardless of the beauty ideals these girls fit; some are bullied for being too pretty and others are antagonized for *not* fitting those ideals. It's all objectifying.

So much research points to the fact that we all walk around with implicit, and often explicit, bias toward others. Weight bias is one glaring example. Women are particularly stigmatized across multiple sectors due to their weight, including employment, education, media, and romantic relationships, among others. In a classic study performed in the 1950s, ten- and eleven-year-olds from varying social, economic, and racial/ethnic backgrounds from across the US were shown six images of children and asked to rank them in the order of which child they "liked best." The six images included what the researchers described as a "normal" weight child, an "obese" child, a child using a wheelchair, a child using crutches and a leg brace, a child with just one hand, and another with a facial difference. Across all samples, the child considered "obese" was ranked last. We argue that a fear and hatred of fat isn't some natural, innate way of being; instead, it is learned and relearned from countless sources throughout our lives.

One of the ways we learn and pass on those biases and ideals comes from parents, caretakers, and guardians, who play a major role in the way children learn about objectification and process their own feelings toward their bodies. Deborah Tannen, a linguistics professor who wrote the book *You're Wearing That? Understanding Mothers and Daughters in Conversation,* identified the three most common sources of friction in mother-daughter conversations as hair, clothes, and weight. Beauty, beauty, and beauty.

Her research describes the mother's desire to protect versus the daughter's desire for approval, which lays the foundation for conflict, shame, and appearance fixation. The well-meaning mother giving advice is driven by a desire to protect her daughter from mean comments and judging eyes, but she has also internalized objectifying, demeaning beauty ideals as "expected" and "necessary." She may believe her daughter is a reflection of herself and want to "correct" in her daughter what she sees as flaws in her own appearance. The approval-seeking daughter takes offense, feeling body shame, anxiety, anger, and sadness. The bond between mother and daughter chips away each time this pattern repeats itself.

The parenting dynamic is more complicated when mothers in particular, or other loved ones or close people in positions of authority, have internalized the belief that the look of their bodies is their most important asset and their responsibility to meticulously maintain. Their example can unintentionally pull their children into the dangerous waters of objectification. This belief shows up in negative self-talk, constant restricting and dieting, exercising for weight control or to make up for "bad" food choices, and seeing their children's appearances as reflections of themselves. All of these actions, whether acknowledged aloud or performed quietly, can pull young children right into the water, and then farther out, into stronger currents and more dangerous waves, by providing a pattern for how they should relate to their own bodies.

One young woman told us about a moment at age sixteen that stuck in her mind, saying, "My mom was helping me buy a swimsuit online. Trying to figure out what size to order, she started taking my measurements. Next thing I knew, she started measuring herself as well and began comparing my 16-year-old body to her 40-year-old body. I quickly began to feel self-conscious as she would ecstatically announce her measurements were the same as mine."

A 2016 study in the *Journal of Clinical Child and Adolescent Psychology* on five- to seven-year-old girls and their mothers revealed what our own lived experiences often make clear: when mothers and their young daughters are put together in front of a mirror, girls emulate how their mothers talk about their bodies. If mom disparages her body, daughter will say equally degrading things about her own body. In the experiment, the mothers were asked to describe their bodies from head to toe. One group had to say only negative things and the other group only positive things. Marisol Perez, one of the lead researchers of the study, said some of the women couldn't find anything kind or redeeming to say about themselves. And what mothers said rang loudly in their daughters' ears. "There was not a single child who did not change their response after hearing their mother say something, either in the positive or negative direction," Perez, an associate professor of psychology at Arizona State University, told the *Atlantic*. "The mother who said she liked her hair, the child echoed. The mother who said she didn't like something, ditto."

In a world that revolves around objectification, we see bodies —our own and others'—as things to be admired and appraised and controlled. In our everyday interactions, we cut down others' body images, reinforce and remind each other of our objectifying environment, police each other's bodies, and get pulled or pull others deeper into the waters of objectification with our words and actions. When we focus on others' looks, not only are we perpetuating a culture of objectification, we are also being divided against each other. We aren't really seeing each other — our friends, sisters, daughters, colleagues, even strangers — as full, complete people irrespective of physical appearance. We often feel like we're competing with other women — including our loved ones — for resources like love, beauty, and validation, even though these things aren't actually limited. These actions and experiences become normal, unquestioned parts of life when we see each other in such limited ways. When we are able to see more in each other, we can unite instead of divide.

Body Compliments

Even when we feel united with other girls and women and our interactions with each other are free from the divisions caused by competitiveness and self-comparison, we still make things difficult for each other. Sometimes, when we're side by side in the sea of objectification, we make comments intended to be kind or helpful about each other's appearance. We do this in the ways we greet each other with a compliment like "You look so tiny!" or "Looking hot!" It happens when a friend or celebrity you follow posts a picture online and you post a comment like "I'm so jealous you lost the baby weight so fast!" or "You look amazing. You have to tell me what you're doing!"

You might not hear anything wrong in those comments, and interpret and intend them only as harmless expressions of kindness, support, acknowledgment, and positivity. The problem with these compliments and conversations that seem so harmless on the surface is that they perpetuate the idea that we are most valued for our looks and always being evaluated accordingly. Any comment about appearance functions as a little splash —a friendly, nonaggressive, well-intentioned splash—that nevertheless instantly directs your attention back to the waters of objectification, where you are defined by how you appear over anything else.

When they're about bodies, constant kind words can actually be *un*kind, as they serve to reinforce beauty as the foremost asset you have to offer the world. A girl or woman scrolling through Instagram every day, as millions of us do, is pummeled with comments on her friends', sisters', and favorite influencers' photos about each inch of their bodies: "Your booty looks 🔥 🔥 🔥 🔥 in those leggings!" *Splash.* "I'm in love with your hair!" *Splash.* "Will you do a makeup tutorial?" *Splash.* "#bodygoals." *Splash.* "Did you lose weight?" *Splash.* These "kind" words reinforce the value and importance of appearance, which triggers people to be hyperfocused on their own parts. This perpetuates a culture of objectification in which most of us are complicit without even knowing it.

Even compliments we receive from people we love can reinforce our need to vigilantly monitor ourselves. Consider how looks-based compliments impact you: A regular visit to your aunt's house can throw you into the downward pull of self-objectification when she says, "Your new lashes look so good!" or "Your skin looks so clear!" *Splash, splash.* Because it's too easy to make the jump to thinking, "Ugh, she noticed these lash inserts so fast that my natural lashes must have looked terrible! Reminder to self to make an appointment to get them redone in a month." Or "My skin must normally be so awful when she sees me if that's what she noticed," while you make plans to remember to wear makeup next time you see her. Once you realize that these well-meaning compliments don't actually boost your body image, you are equipped to make some changes to how you validate people.

Too often, the compliments we receive about our bodies revolve around the ways women have been taught to exist in our world—by taking up as little space as possible. When a woman loses weight, whether on purpose or due to illness or trauma, weight-loss comments are often inescapable. These comments reinforce the lie that thinner is always best, healthiest, and worth any illness, trauma, depression, or insufficient access to food that causes you to achieve it. When you've lost weight, regardless of the reason, well-meaning people will often say, "Wow, you've never looked better!" One woman told us, "When I was young, everyone called me 'Skinny Minnie' and praised me for being so tall and slender. I felt like I had to maintain that, and I recognized that this was something that was valued by others." *(Splash.)*

There's no doubt that much of the time comments like that feel fantastic. It's nice to be acknowledged! If weight loss was something you were intentionally seeking and you're feeling good about it, that little splash when others acknowledge your changing body is refreshing. But there are some factors and scenarios in which this feedback system validating weight loss and thinness for all does some real damage. It is critical to consider that what one person might think of as positive acknowledgment for getting smaller can spark and reinforce feelings of body anxiety in others — little others, vulnerable others, struggling others.

Comments centered on weight loss can be hurtful, as shown by these examples from real women we spoke to during our research and who shared their experiences with us on social media:

"I remember being in the ER, waiting to be preapproved for admission to an eating disorder unit. A nurse who came in to check my vitals had to use a pediatric cuff because my arm was so thin. She commented, 'I wish I was as thin as you!' Apparently she didn't know why I was in the ER. I replied, 'Well, I'm here because I need to be admitted for an eating disorder. So, no you don't.' She was silent after that."

"[After losing weight all] of this new attention found me wanting to be sure to hide my flabby arms (because losing lots of weight leaves a lot of skin) and saggy boobs (because I'd been either pregnant and/or nursing for the last five years). And no matter how wrong I knew it was, I couldn't help but think to myself, If people think I look good now, they'll really think I look good if I lose 20 more pounds . . ."

"Last year, four months after giving birth, I began focusing on getting healthy, eating right, and exercising.

Here's what I was not happy about: the fact that every-one I had ever met all of a sudden felt it was appropriate to comment on my physical appearance. Casual acquaintances felt like it was perfectly reasonable to start asking me about my weight and size. Family members would tell me how good I looked now, and I couldn't help but feel bad for me from a year ago, who I had loved, but apparently everyone else was thinking could be a lot better. I have never felt so uncomfortable in my own skin in my life. I — a woman who has always felt infinitely more defined by my thoughts and humor than by a number on a scale — suddenly felt very self-conscious about everything."

"I lost a considerable amount of weight, and suddenly strangers, acquaintances, and also some friends treated me differently. At first it felt kind of good, but when reality hit, it became sad. Since then, I try my best not to comment on peoples' weight, whether they gain or lose it."

"When I lost weight and became super slim, men suddenly became super helpful and polite, and women approached me more openly. When I'm plus-size, I become completely invisible and unworthy of help or attention. It's actually ridiculous and shows how deeply shallow many people are."

"I lost 25 pounds in less than 2 months due to stress and grief over my brother's death. Wow, the compliments I got, and the 'how did you do it?'"

"It's happened to me twice—first time I was in hospital for a week and couldn't eat solids for about 3 weeks. Lost a ton of weight, got all the compliments. Second time I'd just come out of a long-term relationship and the stress meant I couldn't eat a full meal without feeling sick, so I didn't eat. I exercised too much as well, and yet everyone told me how healthy I looked and how much better I looked."

"I lost a bunch of weight due to illness and my doctor was one of the first to say, 'You look great!' even though she knew how sick I was. Friends and coworkers, same story. Just don't make comments about people's appearance. If you're truly concerned, ask them how they are or how their health is."

"I have ulcerative colitis. One particularly bad flare saw me drop 5kg in 5 days, around 15kg in total. I was terribly unwell and rail thin, and it wasn't an uncommon statement to hear 'I wish I could lose weight that quickly and easily.' I now carry a few extra kg than usual—I think of it as my 'insurance' in prep for future flares!"

"I was a stay-at-home mom pregnant with my third. My husband of 7 years decided that the responsibility of home ownership and a wife and kids just wasn't 'fun' anymore. Our divorce was finalized when I was 5 months pregnant. Instead of gaining weight, I lost 25 lbs through the course of my pregnancy. I would get comments like 'Oh you look so good' and 'You've

> really done well not gaining weight,' and after the baby,
> I continued to lose weight. When I would tell people I
> was divorced, they were shocked because they were too
> busy complimenting me and asking me how I lost the
> baby weight."

Dress Codes and Objectification

When you see someone as a body first and a person second, you are likely to be tempted to regulate and monitor that person's body, which often happens at their expense. Girls' and women's bodies in particular are often seen as threats to onlookers because they are perceived to be distracting and provocative. We most often see this play out in the dress-code and "modesty" enforcement that takes place in schools and churches, and in the social norms that are created in those institutional cultures. Of course, the bodies themselves don't directly, actively cause any harm, and may or may not be intended to do any distracting or provoking, but the viewing of them is said to be harmful, so the bodies are held responsible. Those perceived as doing the threatening are almost exclusively female, while those supposedly being provoked are almost exclusively male.

Society sets rules to regulate the ways female bodies are allowed to appear with the intention of protecting the male bodies and minds that apparently need to be externally (and not internally) controlled. This starts young. We measure hemlines and shoulder straps. We ask girls to kneel on the floor to see where their skirt hits or lift their arms to see if any midriff is revealed. We enforce dress codes that outline every female part that needs to be covered. We do our own modesty policing in the whispers of "Look how much of her legs is showing" and "You can see her stomach when she lifts up her arms!" This veiled objectification starts very young.

Girls learn the most important thing about them is how they look.

Boys learn the most important thing about girls is how they look.

Girls look at themselves.

Boys look at girls.

Girls are held responsible for boys looking at them.

Girls change how they look.

Boys keep looking.

The problem isn't how girls look.

The problem is how everyone looks at girls.

Having their bodies and clothing be regulated or reprimanded is one way girls get pushed into the waters of objectification. The push comes when we are asked to change our clothes and cover more skin at camp since there are men nearby. It comes in church when we are taught to dress modestly in order to avoid being a "stumbling block" for the young men who struggle with tempting thoughts. It happens at school when we're asked to call our parents to bring a sweater or given clothing that obscures our shape after a complaint from a fellow student who felt distracted by our presence.

The push sends us right into the waves and currents of objectification. Even if it wasn't malicious, the revelation that our bodies are being appraised by others and having effects we weren't aware of is a shock that separates us from ourselves. We suddenly exist outside ourselves. We start trying to figure out how to understand and control our bodies and the effects they have on others. For children, adolescents, and young teens, this is often a startling wake-up call to the realities of life in the sea of objectification and the outsized role our bodies play in how we are valued and perceived.

Throughout our lives, as we are regulated and policed by others, we often join in on upholding and enforcing this same policing on others. Two big ways we do this formally in society are through secular dress codes and religious modesty rules. This has been a particularly hot topic over the last few years with a news story popping up every few weeks or so with an egregious example of school dress codes gone awry, or of a girl being kicked out of school or an important event because of one administrator's opinion about her clothing. We have been outspoken for many years about the ways modesty rhetoric and the enforcement of certain one-sided dress codes uphold the sexual objectification of girls and women. For instance, here's a real-life example in the text from a flyer we saw for a "church prom" in the western US:

Boys: *Tie and button-down shirt required. No low-rider pants.*

Girls: *Sleeves should cover the shoulder and top of the arm. No cleavage showing. No bras or bra straps showing through sheer fabrics. No low necklines in the front or*

*back. No open, sheer, bare lace-ups in front or back. No
midriff showing with arms raised while dancing. No tight or
revealing clothes of any kind. No sheer, lacy, or see-through
fabric in areas that should otherwise be covered. Shoulders included. Hems should be no shorter than three-fin-
gers' width above the knee. The back of the dress must
be higher than a bra strap. No low backs. Get your dress
approved via text . . .*

That wasn't even all of it! This ultra-specific list of rules for
girls' dresses and bare minimum requirements for boys illustrates
so much about what the adults in charge fear. Lengthy, over-the-
top, ultra-specific dress codes *for girls only* are based in fear and
anxiety about sex — especially about male sexuality and the feelings female bodies are sure to incite. **But dress codes like these
don't prevent girls from being perceived as sexual objects
— they reinforce it.** They take the focus off of girls and women
as people and hyperfocus on each part of them in need of covering, thus sexualizing those parts or positioning them as inappropriate. Shoulders, knees, backs, stomachs, thighs, underarms, etc.,
are not inherently sexy or sexual. When dress codes demand that
they be covered up, boys learn right alongside girls that those
particular female parts are inappropriate and are, thus, sexually
charged. They also learn that it is normal and appropriate to
objectify girls and women, which is an understanding they will
carry into adulthood.

When girls are policed for dress-code violations and taught to dress modestly to protect others—for example, boys who might be distracted or tempted—they learn and relearn to experience their bodies from a sexualized outside perspective—as objects to be looked at. A young woman becomes her own twenty-four-hour body police, joining the rest of the world in enforcing our culture's arbitrary and unachievable standards of beauty and attractiveness against herself while *also* trying to stay within the lines of "appropriate." Cute but not *too* cute. Sexy but not *too* sexy. In the midst of these unyielding currents and waves of objectification, she is held accountable not only for how she presents herself, but also for how she is perceived by everyone else.

It is especially disheartening when these messages come from churches and organizations that truly care about girls (or *should* truly care about girls), because they are echoing and reinforcing what the larger outside culture constantly tells girls about themselves: they are bodies first and people second. Girls are consistently called out and sent home from school and church and their accompanying events because their attire is deemed inappropriate in often arbitrary ways. Girls with more curvaceous, mature bodies often bear the brunt of dress codes that less developed or less curvy girls don't have to experience.

Modesty is entirely subjective. One person's sophisticated sleeveless blouse is another person's immodest undershirt. One person's comfy, inexpensive, full-coverage leggings are another person's too-hot-for-TV sexy pants. (Obviously, we're referring to definitions of "appropriate" that can vary significantly but still fall within common, legal public attire and fit dress codes for certain venues.) And the context! Oh, the context. Why is a body in leggings objectifiable on the street but not at the gym? Or in a short skirt at dinner but not on a tennis court?

What constitutes "revealing" for one person or family or culture might be fully accepted as "modest" by another person, family, or culture. And women covering up their bodies has no bearing on men's ability to control themselves or respect women. Even in cultures in which women are required to or choose to cover up a great deal, there are still incredibly high incidences of rape and sexual violence. And in some cultures in which clothing is optional, including in some indigenous tribes, rape and sexual violence are reportedly very low.

Every time we teach girls to meticulously cover their bodies in order to protect themselves and to protect men from themselves, we reinforce a view of women as objects. Don't get us wrong, dress codes are often necessary and helpful to ensure everyone is on the same page about what to wear, but they can be guided by mutual respect instead of objectification. (More on how to do this on page 197.)

We see why dress codes can be important, because we live in a world where studies show girls as young as six years old are sexualizing themselves in response to media messages that teach them that being sexy yields rewards. And the fashion industry is markedly gendered, with sexualized, form-fitting clothing common for little girls while boys' clothing allows for movement and function. In a piece written for the *New York Times* on the fashion industry's gender divide, writer Sara Clemence laments the effort it took her to find appropriate clothing for her young daughter that would provide the same pockets, enforced knees, and utilitarian design she could find for her son: "I found girls' sections filled with lightweight leggings, scoop-neck tops, and embellished shoes. I scoured the internet for girls' pants with capacious pockets and reinforced knees, and found maddeningly few options. I eventually realized that, even in an age of female fighter pilots and #MeToo, boys' clothes are largely designed to be practical, while girls' are designed to be pretty . . . It's not just about avoiding skinned knees, but also the subtle and discouraging message that's woven right into girls' garments: *you are dressed to decorate, not to do.*"

The more we teach girls they are here to be looked at, the more we keep them at a disadvantage. The more we value and devalue other women based on how they look and what they're wearing —too fat, too thin, too covered up, not covered up enough—the more we keep them, and ourselves, at a disadvantage. We can't see other women as more than bodies if we're stuck in a mindset of evaluating and patrolling how they might be appearing to others or the effects their appearance might have on others. We offer some positive alternatives to modesty policing on page 197.

Be More Compassionate

Compassion is, by definition, relational. Compassion literally means "to suffer with," which implies a basic mutuality in the experience of suffering. The emotion of compassion springs from the recognition that the human experience is imperfect.

— Kristin Neff, author of *Self-Compassion: The Proven Power of Being Kind to Yourself*

In a culture that too often pits women against each other in competition, recognizing what we have in common — *our common humanity* — can decrease our feelings of isolation and our actual isolation from each other. We can learn to see our experiences, our pain, and our joys as part of the larger human experience rather than seeing them as separating and isolating. Suffering, failure, and inadequacies are part of the human condition. All people — including you — are worthy of care and compassion. As soon as you develop compassion for yourself, your heart is softened to everyone you come in contact with. You begin to see everyone's humanity, which allows you to work in unity instead of competition.

United with Compassion

We would all probably be shocked to know about the sheer number of people who face body shame and who fall short in self-comparison every day — even those you might never imagine feeling that sort of pain. After our speaking engagements, it never fails that some of the most traditionally beautiful women in the room will come up to us and tell us of their deep-seated struggles with body image and the life-sucking burden of trying to maintain their looks and assets that have always brought them the most value and validation. No one is spared.

It is possible to acknowledge the difficulty of navigating the waters of objectification and be more generous in your views of other people and their choices. **You can stop seeing others as competition or threats and instead see allies, friends, and helpers.** You can bond with women you used to judge as too vain, too immodest, too fat, too beautiful. You can take your mom's comment about your body and recognize her internalized objectification without internalizing it yourself. You can see the pain and shame of women being masked by products, procedures, and diets and validate them for more than their "improved" appearances. You can stop seeing other women as objects to be evaluated, sexy threats to your relationship, or alluring distractions to your sons, and instead see all people as full humans with full agency.

If you find yourself tempted to judge someone else or compare yourself to her, especially if she seems to have put a lot of effort into her appearance or sexual appeal, try to shift your perspective with compassion. Instead of making a snap judgment about her character, anxiously wondering if your partner is looking at her, or making a cutting remark about her makeup or surgical "enhancements," remind yourself that she is facing the same objectifying beauty ideals you are. She might be making different decisions than you have, and that's okay. You are in the waters of objectification together, but she isn't a reflection of you. Her beauty work doesn't reflect on you in any way, and isn't a challenge to you to meet the standard she has set. You don't have to look like her or do the same work to feel good or worthy or normal. It's up to you to choose how you will view and value others —as just a collection of parts to be evaluated, or as more than a body.

When you are in a deep dive on Instagram, scrolling through photos of your ex's new partner, and you feel that wave of jealousy and inadequacy brought on by self-comparison, sit with it. Acknowledge what you are doing as you are scrolling through that person's highlight reel and comparing their favorite angles to your least favorite. Really feel and acknowledge that uncomfortable sting you get from self-comparison. Tell yourself something like this: "She is good, and I am good. We are in this together. We aren't in competition for limited resources. I want what is best for her, and I'm sure she'd want the same for me." And then wish her well and put down your phone.

Try to go into any situation with an open heart toward yourself and everyone else, and if you're in a position to open up and share, don't be surprised when your vulnerability is met with total understanding and common experiences. As you open up in whatever way you feel comfortable, you will feel less inclined to judge and compare and compete because you will find community. The common humanity we all share can help us band together and keep each other afloat.

Since our environment makes self-objectification and the constant pursuit of thinness the norm even as it hurts us, watch out for others in need who don't even know they can or should signal for help. A young woman told us, "A coworker of mine stood outside the bathroom one day as I was purging the doughnuts the front desk staff had just given us. When I came out of the bathroom, she kindly confronted me about the issue. It was the first time I had ever spoken to a peer about it. She told me it was unhealthy, and I knew she was right. But I wanted so badly to be thin! I would do anything! Our conversation helped. Therapists helped."

In opening up about your own struggles, you will inevitably attract others whose courage is sparked by your own. You will hear about pain and fear that sounds familiar, but you might also hear about struggles that are hard to understand from people you wouldn't expect. A woman who participated in our studies shared a powerful example of bonding over the trauma of disordered eating with her mom as a teenager. She said, "While growing up, I experienced multiple occasions where my weight was the topic of family conversations. As I grew older I became obsessed with the way I looked. I was a freshman in college when my mom discovered I was making myself throw up. It was then she told me of her lifelong struggle with bulimia. Since then, my mom and I have both fought to get healthier and happier. Together we have strived to make ourselves happy and healthy, fighting to break the cycle so that one day if I happen to have a daughter, she won't go through the same difficulties. This was a really great moment for my mom and I."

Many times, moms or other caretakers who haven't healed their own body image issues (or haven't confronted or acknowledged them at all) may inadvertently treat girls in the same way they treat themselves or were treated when they were children. Moms see their young daughters gaining weight (which they should—the average child gains forty pounds during puberty!) and believe that prodding them about what they eat or how they look will help them have happier childhoods and avoid bullying and alienation. In an effort to help their daughters avoid the pain of body shame, they think the solution is to help them keep their bodies small and thin instead of confronting the larger issues of their own fear of fat or weight gain as well as of society's harmful treatment of girls and women in bodies deemed larger than they should be. To individually and collectively heal the next generation of girls' body image issues, we must work to reject these oppressive thin ideals in our own lives instead of turning that divisive view on our daughters, younger sisters, nieces, and friends.

Now that you are more aware of our culture of objectification, the specific forms of compassion you can offer to others might look different than they did before. Before, your go-to form of kindness might have been a splash of praise for someone's weight loss or other aspects of her appearance. Now, think about how you can validate others for more than their bodies or beauty, digging deeper into their humanity. Before, you might have gently pushed the girls and women in your life with modesty policing comments or actions, thinking you were simply offering good advice or abiding by the rules. Now, it's time to rethink your ideas about modesty standards and dress codes in ways that prioritize compassion over fear or judgment. Before, you might have pulled your friends, sisters, or daughters into the waters of objectification through your own example or been pulled in by your own parents or caretakers. Now, it's time to reconsider the ways your personal choices and interactions could be centered in consideration and love. Your humanizing, compassionate view of others can give you the ability to find connection despite the divisions caused by objectification.

Better Than Body Compliments

Our little splashes toward each other in the form of body comments are often friendly and well intended, but they often reflect exactly what we have been taught to value in ourselves and others: smallness, thinness, youth, and all the other narrow ideals about beauty. When girls and women are bullied because of their looks, or when another viral trend like the "Am I Ugly" videos takes the internet by storm, it is easy to react with an immediate, "You're not ugly! You are beautiful!" Our ideas about beauty are so incredibly intertwined with our ideas about self-esteem that we often don't realize the necessity of separating the two. But assuring someone that she is beautiful will not protect her from the pain of being called ugly. If you give looks-based comments the power to build people up, you reinforce their power to tear people down. Continuing to focus on someone's looks — even in positive ways — uses the same framework and logic that makes appearance-based insults so lethal. *The truth is, when we stop giving beauty the power to make us, we take away its power to break us.*

To help a girl's self-worth and help her build resilience for future beauty-related disappointments, teach her she is *more* than beautiful. Don't just reassure her that her body looks great. Teach her that her body *is* great. Don't cover her pain with a beauty Band-Aid. Instead, help her see what she can learn from her pain to be stronger, more compassionate, and more driven to alleviate suffering in the world. Tell her who she really is—generous, observant, smart, loving, curious, energetic, creative, articulate, compassionate, talented, etc. Compliment her in ways that remind her she is *more:* "I see the way you include those kids who want to play. You are so kind and compassionate." Or "You are an incredible artist. You have a gift that speaks to people's hearts." Or anything else that helps her see that her purposes extend far beyond how well she decorates the earth. When she can find her many purposes, her body won't be her go-to source for value or acceptance.

Similarly, what if someone you care about calls herself or someone else "fat" or asks if you think she's fat? Even if it goes against your natural inclination, try to avoid showing any disapproval, shock, or other negative reaction. We have to take the stigma out of the perfectly normal and natural diversity of body shapes and sizes, including and especially for those who have been disparaged and derided as being too big or too different. For young kids and adults alike, we can learn to respond without putting a value on fat. It's not good or bad, it's not mean or nice, it just *is.* For kids, say something like, "Our fat keeps us warm, protects our insides, and our bodies use it as energy. Isn't that cool?" or "You are so lucky your body has fat on it—that means you're alive and well." Talk openly about how some bodies have more fat than others, for lots of different reasons, and that how much fat a person has on their body doesn't tell you anything else about them, including how healthy they are, how strong they are, how nice or smart or successful or happy or lovable or anything else.

Be aware that the moment you respond to anyone, child or adult, calling someone "fat" by telling her "that's not nice" or "she's not fat—she is beautiful!" you are setting up "fat" as the opposite of "beautiful" and "good" and "worthy," which makes sense when so many of the cultural messages we receive throughout our lives do just that. However, it isn't true or helpful. We can counteract that, slowly but surely, in our own lives by being advocates and defenders and celebrators of body diversity in all its forms. The most important work you can do to buoy up the body images of younger generations is to be aware of your own biases and prejudices about fat, cellulite, stretch marks, weight gain, and anything else you tend to despise in your own body and others'. You need to not only hide those harmful biases and self-deprecating tendencies from your kids, but also actively show them what you appreciate in yourself and others. Show them what you value in the ways you speak about your own body and others' —even celebrities'. Do you admire her strength, talents, fashion choices, words, or actions? Say it. Skip size and weight comments entirely, about yourself and anyone else. When we begin to see women as more than bodies, the look of those bodies becomes one of the least interesting parts about them.

Much of the time, we talk about each other's appearances because we're trying to be kind. There's nothing wrong with a nice compliment. But we want to raise a big red flag here to say our culture's obsession with thinness and physical "perfection" has warped our ideas of how to view and value each other. When our first, natural instinct is to praise a woman's appearance over anything else about her, we clearly have a limited view of her and what she needs. If we really believe we are more than bodies to be looked at, we can work on advocating for this message in small, powerful ways. Looks-based compliments can sometimes be really nice, but we can all dig deeper—especially for someone you see regularly or know on a level deeper than the surface. Instead of telling her, "You look amazing!" tell her, "You *are* amazing!" Obviously, you should get more specific whenever possible. What have you observed in her character, talents, actions—or really, anything other than how she appears—that you find admirable or worth acknowledging?

You can even reframe those body-based comments from your loved ones that used to send you shame spiraling. "You've lost weight and look incredible" or "You could use a little meat on those bones" or "Why don't you wear makeup? You look so pretty when you put a little effort in" can be an opportunity to open up and bond. Consider responding with something like "I know you mean that as a compliment, but I'm working on my body image and that means I'm trying to find my value beyond my looks. I could really use a reminder that I'm worth more than how I appear!" or "Thanks! And you just reminded me that I've actually set a goal to validate people for more than their bodies. Do you want to try this out with me? It's hard at first, but so worth it to help people see how amazing they are for more than their looks." You could also use it as an opportunity to see how they are doing, because their comments generally reveal what they are fixated on or worried about in their own life. Responding by simply asking questions like "How are you feeling?" "What have you been up to?" or "What can I do for you?" can take the focus off of you and get somewhere deeper with your loved one.

Moms, caretakers, and loved ones can and should step in to mediate looks-based comments directed at young girls when possible. If a girl you are close to is often complimented for her beauty or thinness or other aesthetic appeal, we recommend being firm and explicit about avoiding these comments whenever possible. When appropriate, it can be helpful to illuminate your reasons for avoiding body talk. Be real with people. Tell them you've struggled to value yourself as more than a body and you're working really hard to make sure you can keep up your progress and teach the ones in your care that they are valuable for more than how they appear. If a loved one has struggled with disordered eating or self-consciousness, consider sharing that with the commenter (if your loved one approves) and explaining that you are working to avoid those problems in any way you can. If a girl in your life is explicitly complimented for how thin she is, try something along the lines of, "We're actually working together to get rid of the 'thinner is better' mind-set since we've seen how much it has hurt people." Let them know you are working to notice and compliment people on more than their outsides, and trying to value more in yourself too.

If you don't feel comfortable making a real statement, however gently, you can work to change the conversation to illuminate the fact that the girl is more than her body. Pivot to say something like "She is feeling strong after all that swimming!" or "Did you know she has been learning Spanish?" or "[Insert child's name], do you want to tell them about the book you've been reading?" You don't want to call people out in a way that might be embarrassing in public. Lexie has taught her daughter to respond to all the comments about how cute she is by saying, "Thanks! And I'm smart, too!" Not only is it adorable, but it also drives home a perfectly appropriate and enlightening point. Some people will be offended and defensive regardless of how kindly you share your perspective—and in those cases, be compassionate about the comfort zone they're coming from—but some will be able to graciously take your note and make changes.

When you consider what you value in other people, whether kids or adults, those things can show up in your compliments. Try something like "I heard that comment you gave in class, and I thought it was so smart I wrote it down. You are such a wordsmith." Or "You are so great at talking to people and going out of your way to make people feel comfortable and acknowledged. You are such a good example to me." Or "I saw you post on Facebook about that political campaign you are volunteering for. You are such a powerhouse! Tell me what got you into this." These are the kinds of comments that hit home—they are meaningful and can't be brushed off with "Oh thanks, but this is just good shapewear!"

In response to this push against beauty-focused compliments, we are often asked, "Should I talk to other women about their looks at all?" We fully recognize that beauty-related compliments are often nice and welcomed. Still, use your best judgment while keeping in mind the little splash you might be sending toward whoever you want to praise. It might be an unwelcome reminder to think about her appearance, or it might be the only thing she ever hears compliments about when she would instead really love to be acknowledged for her work, kindness, character, or other aspects of her humanity.

Where we *do* absolutely draw the line is on body-size-related comments. Just don't do it.

Let's try a pop quiz: If you know someone who has lost weight, but you don't know how or why she did it, what do you do?

A: Compliment, compliment, compliment! The more praise about her fab new bod, the better.

B: Don't say anything in person, but next time you see her on Instagram or Facebook, throw down a little "You look so skinny!" on a couple pics to let her know you noticed.

C: Talk about anything else besides her looks. Her job. Your lunch. That dog walking by. Anything else. Ask her how she is doing, feeling—anything.

This might feel like a trick question. All compliments are nice, right? We know the reality is a bit more complicated than that. Think of it this way: Most of us fluctuate in weight for all kinds of reasons. If you've lost a noticeable amount of weight, it is almost guaranteed you have had lots of well-meaning friends and acquaintances compliment you with those types of reinforcing "You've never looked better!" comments. And you might really believe that and really love hearing it. But what we know is that research shows the vast majority of us will gain most or all of the weight back again within a few short years or less. And when those compliments stop, it is so easy to let body shame sink in that tells us we're valuable and attractive and worthy only when we are thinner and take up less space.

From Lexie: Last year after a two-week bout with the flu that caused me to lose weight, one of my coworkers noticed and would explicitly compliment me each day. In an effort to gently help her understand that her comments weren't welcome, I said, "I know you're trying to be nice, but here's the thing: I've lost weight because I've been sick, and it hasn't been fun! I guarantee you I'm about to gain this weight back, and when I do, you're going to stop complimenting me. That won't be fun for either of us!" and then I laughed and she did, too. But she got the point, and I haven't received a weight-based compliment since.

Seeing more in each other requires us to halt harmful, objectifying body policing and replace it with conversations, questions, and compliments that take us beyond the objectifying waters we know so well. Ask people about life. Ask them how they are feeling. Redirect the conversation. Acknowledge other aspects of their humanity. Give them space to open up to you if they want to. As we learn to truly accept and value body diversity and destigmatize fatness, we give ourselves the space to be considerate of others' full humanity in the ways we talk to and about them.

All along the way, we need to check our own biases by learning about, acknowledging, and consciously challenging them — whether they are about others' bodies and faces or our own. In her essay "La Güerra," Chicana feminist scholar Cherríe Moraga writes, "Without naming the enemy within ourselves and outside us, no authentic, non-hierarchical connection among oppressed groups can take place." This opens us to what she calls "frightening questions," such as, "How have I internalized my own oppression? How have I oppressed?" As both the oppressors and the oppressed, we can think deeply and critically about these questions to help us determine when we are perpetuating the prejudices and objectification around us and when we are working to combat them.

Dress Codes for the Wearer, Not the Watcher

As you build compassion and recognize our common humanity in an objectifying culture, your views on modesty and how it is enforced—through dress codes or through unspoken cultural norms—might shift. Your inclination to police others' bodies might decline. We hope it does. How everyone else sees girls and women and feels about their bodies and clothes is less important than how girls and women see themselves and how *they* feel in their bodies and clothes. This is about recognizing and valuing the agency and humanity of all people—those being looked at and those doing the looking.

We understand the desire to clearly articulate a dress code for young women, who are slammed with messages telling them their value lies in their sexual appeal above all else. But hyperspecific dress codes for girls don't help that cause, and might do more harm than good by inadvertently sexualizing young women as a collection of inappropriate body parts to be hidden.

The people who wrote the dress code we shared on page 179, and the people who write many dress codes like it, are most often well-meaning, good people. We want to help people channel those good intentions into more effective means of communicating about dress codes, modesty, and bodies in general. By rethinking how they approach dress codes, schools and churches are well positioned to encourage girls to *be more* by teaching them how to understand and seek their value outside of sexual appeal and their appearance. After all, lots of churches preach some pretty nice things about the worth of souls and the source of that great love and power to help individuals. Schools are the perfect place to teach critical thinking and media and cultural literacy skills to help students question the messages they receive about how people are valued and who is oppressed and hurt by those messages.

A constructive dress code prioritizes how girls and women feel in their own bodies and clothing. Not how others feel about them, not how others see them, not even how they visually see themselves—but how they internally *feel* in their clothing and in their bodies. As adults and young women, we can help girls and women have compassion for themselves by teaching them to consciously consider the ways clothing affects their own self-perceptions and self-consciousness, rather than the ways others might or might not perceive them. For example, we could help them become conscious of and critical of the ways we've been taught to view and value ourselves as objects to be looked at, and of the ways this thinking might influence how clothes are designed and marketed to us, as well as influence which clothes we choose to wear.

It is okay and natural to like being looked at, and even to like attention from others for our looks. The complications come when our awareness and hopes of being looked at become distracting and hinder our focus, happiness, and health—as so much research confirms they do. Dress code or no dress code, it's important to remain conscious of the role our clothing plays in holding us back mentally. Studies on self-objectification show us that wearing body-baring and tight clothing leads to greater states of self-objectification, body shame, body dissatisfaction, and negative mood. What this tells us (and what our own experience tells us is a no-brainer) is that when you wear clothing that is especially revealing or emphasizes your body, you become very self-aware of those parts that are most visible and potentially being looked at. You self-objectify and are in a near-constant state of sucking in, posing just right, adjusting your clothing, and fixating on how you might look.

Research shows that finding a level of comfortable coverage from clothing—which will absolutely vary from person to person since comfort is entirely subjective—can be an important tool in safeguarding yourself from self-objectification. This benefit of less body-conscious attire (as defined by the wearer, not the viewer) can be significant for those who fixate on their appearance. On an individual level, think about making clothing choices that prioritize your own comfort, experience, and expression rather than your sexual appeal alone. Sure, your sexual appeal can be part of your personal expression, but when it is the driving force in how you express yourself, you are prone to be worried less about yourself and more about how others perceive you. Which clothes in your closet or drawers right now make you feel your most comfortable and least preoccupied with your appearance? Which clothes leave you constantly adjusting and monitoring yourself? If you are a parent, ask your daughters (and other loved ones) to consider those questions often and make decisions with that in mind. Our success and well-being hinges on how engaged and present we are able to be, and clothing can help or hinder that success.

If you are in a position of power or setting dress codes for other people: Understand what is often really at the root of our desires to police girls' clothing—fear and anxiety about sex and a wish to protect boys from the feelings that female bodies are sure to incite. So much talk of modesty includes the effect women's and girls' clothing choices have on males, but we suggest leaving the viewers out of the dress code conversation. If you are teaching the girls in your lives that the primary objective of modesty is to keep themselves covered so boys and men don't think sexual thoughts about them, then you are teaching girls they are responsible for other people's thoughts and that they are primarily sexual objects in need of covering. We can never be clothed perfectly enough to ensure everyone perceives us the way we *intend* to be perceived. **We have very little control over what other people think when they look at us.**

This isn't a call to abolish all dress standards in every setting. This is a call to create them and enforce them with compassion, consideration, and equality. A well-written dress code can rein-force personal accountability for everyone's appropriate dress, guided by uniform instructions and unilateral (but sensitive) en-forcement for everyone—not just the female ones, not just the especially curvy ones, not just the ones whom the boys might be "distracted by," and not arbitrarily enforced based on any one person's fleeting opinion about any one student or about female bodies in general. If you are creating a dress code, avoid rules that unnecessarily deconstruct girls into collections of body parts to be covered. Instead, think of how they can reinforce personal ac-countability for everyone, guided by uniform instructions about what constitutes appropriate dress for all involved.

Gender-neutral standards can be freeing for everyone. You want everyone to be covered from armpits to fingertips? Great. Shoulders to knees? Great. And in a formal school or church event setting, like a dance, where girls are met with many more options for what to wear than boys generally are, we suggest it might be time to stop requiring girls to wear dresses or skirts. We put them in a real bind when they have to conform to female standards of fashion and then face the added burden of spending incredible amounts of time, money, and energy to find something they feel good in that also fits the dress code. And finally, we rec-ommend letting kids weigh in on the dress standards they'll be held to—what they think is reasonable, appropriate, and accept-able. It might help to listen.

When you are tempted to provide a thorough checklist of what girls can and can't wear, ask yourself what fears are behind your hesitation to lighten up on the dress code? Do you think teens are more likely to have sex if their midriffs or bra straps are exposed at school? That is probably not true. A few extra inches of fabric likely won't stand in their way if that's their decision. Let's talk openly about sex and the pressures young people feel to engage in sexual relationships, whether they're emotionally and mentally ready or not. Are you worried that a boy at school might see the outline of a girl's bum in those leggings, or see down her low-cut shirt, and be distracted? He might. He should get a handle on that and learn how to focus in the face of distractions, because girls and women will never be invisible. He will have a better life if his success doesn't hinge on the absence of women. Focus on talking to kids about being responsible for their own thoughts and actions. Talk to teens about the shame-free realities of their sexual responses and their responsibilities to act with integrity and respect for others. It can be comforting and empowering for teens and adults to know that we all get to decide for ourselves how we use our brains and bodies, and that we can see all people as full-fledged, thinking, feeling humans no matter how they are dressed or how they act.

A Seattle school district made waves online in 2019 when they implemented a district-wide "inclusive dress policy" to make consistent, equitable rules of dress. Under the new policy, students are required to wear a top and bottom — the only stipulations being that "private parts" are covered — and shoes. Clothing carrying sexually suggestive, libelous, violent, or criminal messaging is off-limits.

The district listed their core values related to student dress as the foundation for the rules in the policy as follows:

- Students should be able to dress and style their hair for school in a manner that expresses their individuality without fear of unnecessary discipline or body shaming;
- Students have the right to be treated equitably. Dress code enforcement will not create disparities, reinforce or increase marginalization of any group, nor will it be more strictly enforced against students because of racial identity, ethnicity, gender identity, gender expression, gender nonconformity, sexual orientation, cultural or religious identity, household income, body size/type, or body maturity;
- Students and staff are responsible for managing their personal distractions; and
- Students should not face unnecessary barriers to school attendance.

We applaud this incredible effort at inclusivity, which is now being used as a model in other schools across the country. If you see a problem with your school's dress code, we recommend reaching out to an administrator at the school or district level who could help you champion a similar solution. Send them Seattle's "Inclusive Dress Policy" or a similar one and the core values they used to drive their decisions, and ask them to consider implementing something similar.

When you recognize others' humanity, including the variables that go into why they are wearing what they are wearing, you will be compelled to err on the side of compassion rather than automatic judgment or discipline. This is true for those under your care or leadership as well as people you pass on the streets or scroll past online. What if our default was to view others with compassion rather than judgment? When you feel inclined to police someone else's clothing, challenge your conscious or unconscious motivations or fears. Are the clothes themselves the actual problem, or is the problem our shared culture of objectification?

In your own life, it is up to you to determine whether a level of modesty, whether culturally or religiously imposed, is something you value and seek to uphold. If you grew up in a religion or society that requires a level of coverage of women's hair or bodies, you get to decide how (or whether) you'd like to incorporate those practices into your life. Consider how your clothing and hair-covering choices impact not only your religious or cultural experiences but also your relationship with your body. Do your choices help or hinder your ability to understand and experience your body as an instrument for your use, not as an ornament to be admired?

It is also important to keep in mind that people's individual reasons for choosing to dress modestly or according to certain personal or religious codes might not have anything to do with preventing or protecting themselves from objectification. Our judgments about women's choices in clothing are, again, a symptom of our cultural tendency to objectify and evaluate women based on how they present their bodies and faces. No one questions boys and men for the skin they do or do not show. Can we give girls and women that same freedom from assumptions and judgment, whether they choose to observe religious modesty traditions or not?

What all of this boils down to is our challenge to prioritize how girls and women feel in their own bodies and clothing, rather than how others see them. To consider, and help others consider, the ways clothing affects our self-perceptions and self-consciousness, rather than the ways others might or might not perceive us. To treat others with respect, regardless of how they are dressed or how they look.

In the end, compassion will unite us. When we can learn to see ourselves and everyone else as more than a collection of parts to be seen, we can see our true humanity, in all its complexity. We can bond with people we used to write off as unworthy of our attention because of their looks. We can unite in vulnerability as we name our pain and help others see their value beyond their appearance. We can reduce the underlying tension we feel with people who comment on our bodies by calling it out and helping them see and say more. We can band together to combat objectification — to identify it, uproot it, and replace it with opportunities to rise with resilience together. We aren't in this alone. We can make it to a better destination in partnership with each other.

5

Reclaiming Health and Fitness for Yourself

- How do you determine whether a person is healthy or fit?
- Do you consider yourself healthy or fit?
- Do you want to make any changes to your health? If so, what kinds of changes do you want to make?

See More in Your Health

The phobia about fatness and the preference for thinness have not, principally or historically, been about health.
— Sabrina Strings, *Fearing the Black Body: The Racial Origins of Fat Phobia*

In the media and in our own goals and conversations, health and fitness are frequently described and portrayed in terms of appearance: weight, dress size, measurements, body mass index, whether a body looks "toned," "firm," or "sleek," etc.— so much so that our culture's definitions of beauty and health are pretty much inseparable. Our skewed and warped body image maps have too often pointed us toward destinations of *looking* healthy and fit rather than *feeling* or *being* healthy or fit.

This showed up in our research, too. When our study participants were initially asked to define health and fitness, about 40 percent of their answers included appearance-focused terms. One woman defined it this way: "I don't think it is any specific measurement or weight necessarily, but whatever those measurements need to be to achieve a healthy heart, blood pressure, and activity level. I also think that when those things are achieved, the look of my body will be its best look—nice fit curves, without excess 'hang-over.'" When asked if she considers herself healthy or fit, another woman said, "Well, sort of. I exercise often and try to eat healthy, but I'm not super thin. I'm trying to do Weight Watchers. I attend exercise classes on a regular basis and am training for several races, including Ragnar [a long-distance relay] and a half marathon."

We weren't surprised to discover that most of the women in our research who felt negatively toward their bodies also tended to judge their own health in terms of their appearance. And once again, those who judged their health according to appearance-focused body ideals almost always felt ashamed of their bodies. ***Just like it is incredibly difficult to feel positively about your body when you're judging it based on looks, it is incredibly difficult to feel positively about your health when you are judging it based on looks.*** Those looks are wildly hard to achieve and have nothing to do with health! It's no wonder so many women feel like health is beyond their reach. When asked whether they considered themselves healthy or fit, the women in our research who felt ashamed of their bodies overwhelmingly believed health and fitness were either entirely out of reach or could be reached only with extreme deprivation and self-sacrifice.

One woman in our research who felt negatively about her body overall described how she was currently working as an aerobic instructor, taking weight-lifting classes, hiking regularly, and exercising daily, plus trying "very, very hard to make healthy eating choices" every day. However, she did not feel like she could describe herself as healthy or fit because of her strong desire to lose 5 to 10 pounds in order to reach her "target weight according to the BMI." Another said, "I do consider myself healthy and fit, but I don't think I have met my potential, because I would like to lose about 10 to 15 pounds before I would consider myself in 'swimsuit' shape."

This reliance on weight and the body mass index (known as the BMI, which is a person's weight in kilograms divided by the square of their height in meters) showed up in lots of our research participants' definitions of health. When asked if she'd describe herself as healthy or fit, one woman said, "Mostly. I am at the high end of my healthy BMI and want to be rid of some of the excess flab that built up since before I had children. But my blood pressure and other labs indicate that my body is pretty happy with the way things are. I am able to participate in all of the daily activities that I want."

Like this woman making the point that her health seems great despite what her "excess flab" might suggest, many people find that there are better markers of their own good health than simple measurements of fat. World-class athletes and unarguably fit people don't always look like (or weigh like) our cultural ideals for fit bodies, so their performance and their experiences within their own bodies are much better signs of their health than their measurements or reflections. Other ways to evaluate our own health (often with the help of a medical professional) include measuring internal indicators like heart rate, blood pressure, blood sugar, blood lipids, and respiratory fitness. Blood tests can reveal much more about a person's metabolic health than their dress size can.

Even without a doctor or any professional to administer tests or evaluate your results, there are still helpful and effective ways to determine whether you are in good health—keeping in mind that this is a subjective state of being that will differ for each person. Disability, chronic illness, and disease affect people's experiences in their own bodies and their capacity for experiencing good health in huge ways, making it all relative and not entirely within your own control. A huge variety of factors shape your individual experiences with physical health, which makes it impossible to determine one baseline for what constitutes "healthy" for everyone.

Be honest with yourself as you consider your own health *without* focusing on your weight or shape. How do you feel in your daily life? How do you feel when you play with kids, walk down the street, take the stairs instead of the elevator, or go on a hike? Does your body serve you how you want it to? Are you able to do the activities and tasks you want or need to do in your life without getting too winded and struggling through it, or ending up in pain due to lack of cardiovascular fitness or muscle strength?

Are you satisfied with the amount of energy you have on a typical day, or are you more tired and sluggish than you would like? Do you feel generally well, or do you feel that something might be out of balance inside your body — nutritionally, digestively, metabolically, cardiovascularly, or in another way that affects your physical well-being?

Weight and Body Mass Index

For many of us, measuring our weight has become a substitute for measuring our health. But does your weight really correlate with your health in an obvious way? The majority of us have had our weight and height measured at the doctor's office or even on our elementary school report cards, with our body mass index (BMI) reported back to us or our parents, noting whether or not we're in a "healthy" range. Even if a person has no significant complaints of health issues, many doctors will still prescribe weight loss to get her into the "normal" weight range, usually defined by BMI.

One woman told us how her doctor's emphasis on her weight caught her off guard and stuck with her. She said, "Weight and body image haven't ever really been an issue for me, that is, until I got pregnant with my first child. When I got pregnant, I gained more weight, as is normal. I didn't really think much of my weight gain until my doctor made it a point in every appointment to point out how much weight I had gained in the previous month, two weeks, etc. Each appointment I heard something like, 'Wow! You gained 10 pounds this month, you really need to be watching how much you gain' . . . But by all standards, the baby and I were healthy."

This woman went on to say she was very dissatisfied with that doctor — who failed to diagnose her with a serious condition that caused her to swell — and had since found a new one, but the constant attention to her growing body was hard to shake. She said, "Because of [that doctor's] preoccupation with my weight while pregnant, I have developed a preoccupation with my weight while pregnant as well. I am now pregnant with my third child, and find myself saying and thinking things that I shouldn't, but I should celebrate more the wonderful thing that is going on inside my body. I hate that I do this because we are all different people with different body types and I should celebrate those differences and not be jealous of them."

Plenty of research has been done in the last several years on the problems with correlating a person's weight with their health, as well as how ineffective it is to determine someone's healthy weight according to the body mass index. To breeze through just a few issues with the standard BMI chart promoted by the CDC: it doesn't take gender into account despite healthy levels of fat and weight distribution differing greatly between men and women; it is based on a Caucasian standard, though even the World Health Organization has acknowledged the extensive evidence that "the associations between BMI, percentage of body fat, and body fat distribution differ across populations"; it doesn't take age into consideration, so it doesn't allow for weight naturally (and healthily) increasing with age; it doesn't account for body frame or muscle mass, which leads to serious miscalculations of body fat; and Adolphe Quetelet, the French scientist who developed the original height-to-weight ratio that would come to be known as the BMI, intended it for large diagnostic studies on general populations, not individuals. Despite promoting a personal BMI calculator to be used by individuals, the CDC website now states, "BMI can be used for population assessment of overweight and obesity. Because calculation requires only height and weight, it is inexpensive and easy to use for clinicians and for the general public. BMI can be used as a screening tool for body fatness but is not diagnostic."

So why, despite all the evidence against it, do federal health agencies and countless medical professionals continue to rely on BMI for helping individuals understand their health? Because, as the CDC has stated, it is "inexpensive and easy for clinicians and for the general public." It might be misleading and ineffective, but it is cheap and easy. *Yikes.*

Being able to calculate our own BMIs and having our doctors rely on that number to determine whether we're in the healthy range hasn't even put a dent in the much-publicized "obesity crisis" that has been on everyone's radar since the '90s. During that time, weight loss has become the primary goal and the number one prescribed way to improve health. Despite the diet industry's huge profits, the vast majority of people who lose weight — regardless of how they lose it — will gain it all back within two to five years.

In 2007 and then again in 2013, Traci Mann, professor and director of the Health and Eating Lab at the University of Minnesota, along with colleagues Janet Tomiyama and Britt Ahlstrom, conducted a review of every published study of diets conducted with randomized controlled trials that included a follow-up with participants after two years or more. In a 2018 brief of their findings for the American Psychology Association, Mann wrote, "The results were clear. Although dieters in the studies had lost weight in the first nine to 12 months, over the next two to five years, they had gained back all but an average of 2.1 of those pounds. Participants in the nondieting waitlist control groups gained weight during those same years, but an average of just 1.2 pounds. The dieters had little benefit to show for their efforts, and the nondieters did not seem harmed by their lack of effort. In sum, it appears that weight regain is the typical long-term response to dieting, rather than the exception."

Decreasing our weight in any significant way for any significant amount of time is nearly impossible, despite every profit-driven message to the contrary. Our efforts to lose weight by any means necessary often hurt us in the process, leading to cycles of restricting and bingeing, disordered eating, compulsive overexercising, use of unregulated and dubious over-the-counter supplements, and abuse of prescription or illegal drugs.

One woman wrote to us about her own experience suffering under impersonal and rigid measures of health, saying: "I am a recovered bulimic. I battled this disease for 17 years. I was bulimic through some of my pregnancies even. For years, I despised myself . . . I couldn't see my value past what I weighed. Your research on the BMI has lifted a burden from my shoulders like you can't imagine. Even as I have grown in acceptance of myself, I had geared myself up to believe that I would have to love myself in spite of what BMI charts said I should be. Knowing I can disregard them is a freedom I didn't know I could have. I feel like I have taken a deep long breath after breathing through a straw for too long."

One of the scariest facts of all is that in young girls, dieting too often leads to a lifetime of difficulty with food. Starting kids on diets predicts totally different outcomes than what parents expect. In a large study of fourteen- and fifteen-year-olds, dieting was the most important predictor of developing an eating disorder. Those who dieted moderately were five times more likely to develop an eating disorder and those who practiced extreme restriction were eighteen times more likely to develop an eating disorder than those who did not diet. Dieting is associated with increased rates of binge eating in both girls and boys.

At least 30 million people of all ages and genders suffer with eating disorders in the US, and eating disorders have the highest mortality rate of any mental illness, with one person dying every hour as a direct result of an eating disorder, according to the National Association of Anorexia Nervosa and Associated Disorders. These numbers are without a doubt lower than the actual prevalence because so many cases go unreported. The number of *children* — 89 percent female — under age twelve hospitalized due to an eating disorder increased 119 percent from 1999 to 2006. Though a person can develop an eating disorder for any number of reasons, including internal risk factors like genetics and personality type, it is almost always related to external risk factors, like consumption of objectifying media, trauma, and dieting to lose weight.

One of the real difficulties in helping people understand the harms of disordered eating and dieting for weight control or weight loss is that the conventional wisdom says thinness by any means necessary equals good health. Most people believe that ideal body weight is a key factor in anyone's health (in addition to being a key factor in their attractiveness and confidence), and everyone knows the best way to control or lose weight is through reducing the number of calories we take in, right? So, learning to restrict, reduce, count, weigh, monitor, journal, and otherwise fixate on our food from a young age is the healthiest thing to do, right? As shown above, the research says otherwise.

It is completely understandable that so many smart, health-conscious people turn to dieting and find themselves on this punishing cycle. The idea that weight loss is key to health and happiness is so deeply embedded in our world that it's hard to see how profit-driven and false this idea is. In a *New York Times* op-ed, novelist Jessica Knoll wrote, "I called this poisonous relationship between a body I was indoctrinated to hate and food I had been taught to fear 'wellness.' This was before I could recognize wellness culture for what it was—a dangerous con that seduces smart women with pseudoscientific claims of increasing energy, reducing inflammation, lowering the risk of cancer and healing skin, gut and fertility problems. But at its core, 'wellness' is about weight loss. It demonizes calorically dense and delicious foods, preserving a vicious fallacy: Thin is healthy and healthy is thin."

This conflation of thinness and weight loss as "wellness" by industries that profit from it reached peak ridiculousness when Weight Watchers rebranded as simply "WW," with the tag line "Wellness That Works for Every Body." Their famous group weigh-ins are now called "wellness check-ins." Clever. The words *diet* and *weight loss* may be out of fashion in many circles, but their reign as the most important factors in people's ideas about health has not ended. Regardless of how these appearance-focused ideals are packaged, we can all learn to see through the illusions and see more in our health than the outsider's perspective we've adopted to evaluate ourselves. ***Just like we need to redefine beauty in ways that are better for our health, we need to redefine*** **health** ***in ways that have nothing to do with*** **beauty.**

Thinspo and Fitspo

It turns out, losing weight is really hard for most people, and keeping it off is much harder. That doesn't change (and definitely adds to) the pressure people feel to be thin. So we try to encourage and inspire each other, or we seek out and share images of our top body ideals as goals to work toward. In its darkest form, this becomes "thinspiration," or "thinspo." It's an online world of thousands — even millions — of mostly girls and women who share and collect pictures of *very* thin women as inspiration to keep up their eating disorders. It is a saddening and terrifying collection of anonymous internet users banding together to get thin at any cost and "inspiring" themselves to death. Literally. Thousands of girls and women die every year in this pursuit of thin, thinner, thinnest.

Most social media platforms have now banned thinspo, or at least the hashtags that allow people to find it, though that is a constantly changing battleground. After years of campaigns to raise awareness of obvious signs of eating disorders, most people can look at those images of emaciated young girls with flat stomachs, "thigh gaps," and protruding hip bones and recognize that they are dangerous. But the same thinness-focused body pressures that created an environment ripe for thinspo are all over the fitness world as well. No one flinches when the same flat stomachs and "thigh gaps" are attached to a motivating workout slogan and wearing gym clothes. As author Charlotte Hilton Anderson wrote on her blog, *The Great Fitness Experiment*, "Fitspo may be thinspo in a sports bra."

If you are willing to acknowledge that promoting thinspo leads people into danger, you need to also be willing to consider whether your allegiance to similar body ideals in the name of health is a wise move. Start by being on the lookout for how lots of fitness inspiration (aka #fitspo) messages rely on objectification to supposedly motivate or inspire viewers. You can always spot when an objectified idea of fitness is being pushed because the words and images will revolve around aesthetics and will feature only a narrow range of bodies. These messages are hard to avoid, but when you can spot them and see the appearance-fixating strategies at play, they lose some of their power.

Almost all social or advertising-backed media platforms are filled with timely, supposedly motivational advertisements promoting weight loss for *every* occasion: "new year, new you," get your "summer body" or post-breakup "revenge body," fit into a tiny dress on your "big day," or "get your body back" after pregnancy. ***Apparently, it is never not a perfectly festive time to*** *shrink yourself!* While a slogan and image motivating you to get out and move and live and do can be a great thing, so many of these fitspo messages need to be exposed for what they are: objectifying, limiting ideals that keep people focused on their looks as opposed to their health. These images are especially misleading when they conflate "fitness" with body ideals, leading people to think that healthy, fit bodies must necessarily look like the rock-solid, thin-yet-curvy ideals we see everywhere. (Pro tip: they don't. Stand at the finish line of a marathon. Watch the Olympics. Relish the body diversity among world-class athletes and regular, everyday fit people anywhere you turn.)

Sneaky, objectifying fitspo messages almost always feature very, very thin young women who are tanned, oiled up, posed provocatively, and wearing nothing but small swaths of spandex. They are often surgically or digitally enhanced to have the smoothest skin imaginable with little to no body fat except for the meticulously placed and preserved fat in all the "right" places. On video, CGI, bright lighting, and filtered lenses portray bodies with no signs of cellulite, spider veins, ingrown hairs, any hair at all, uneven skin tone, etc. Some of the popular Pinterest-worthy images of the last decade have included slogans like:

- *Suck it up now and you won't have to suck it in later.*
- *Would you rather be covered in sweat at the gym or covered in clothes at the beach?*
- *Girls who are naturally skinny are lucky. Girls who have to fight to be skinny are strong.*
- *Skinny girls look good in clothes. Fit girls look good naked.*

These might seem like a step up from the gross *Nothing tastes as good as skinny feels* thinspo slogans from yesteryear, but they're not a far shot from the same sentiment. They all boil down to "Do whatever it takes to get your body to look like *this,* and then you'll be happy/confident/desirable/worthy of going outside this summer."

Even though we're all familiar with the fit body ideals of the day, keep in mind how much those ideals have changed over time and will continue to change constantly based on what makes companies money—not what makes people healthy. Protruding, rounded backsides paired with teeny tiny waists and thighs that don't touch (*ugh, that insidious "thigh gap"*) wasn't a fitness trend until celebrity influencers made it so. No one outside of a body-building competition was taking "casual" gym selfies in the mirror while twisting and contorting their body to exaggerate their waist-to-hip ratio (and then shrinking or magnifying it further with an app and posting it online). That ain't about fitness ability. That's about sex appeal. It won't last forever, and neither will the next ideal.

Social media has magnified and complicated all of this. Sure, there have been varying fit body ideals forever, but those aspirational images were limited to platforms where you had to seek them out, not surrounding you. Before social media, you'd see idealized bodies on infomercials, magazines, workout tapes, and occasional TV segments, but the body ideals weren't anywhere near as extreme or as cohesive. Now, we see the same rare body types, often augmented by surgical and digital manipulation if not severe malnourishment and dehydration, over and over again in our news feeds. Fitness and beauty influencers with millions of followers, targeted ads across the web, TV and movie stars, and YouTube celebrities represent the same ideals and offer the tricks to achieve them. If you aren't following them, your friends, colleagues, or family members likely are.

When you're so accustomed to monitoring your beauty and performing attractiveness throughout your days and seeing other women in media and in real life doing the same thing, the alternative looks and feels striking. Media representation of female athletes has been notoriously objectifying, focusing on the sexual appeal of their bodies as opposed to their athletic form, and often passively posed, rather than in action. While studying the effects of coverage of female athletes, psychology researcher Elizabeth Daniels sought to find out how objectifying images affected female viewers. She selected images of women that showed sexualized athletes, performance athletes, sexualized models, or nonsexualized models, and asked nearly six hundred participants aged thirteen to twenty-two to complete worksheets measuring self-objectification after viewing certain images from one of the four categories. Those who had viewed sexualized, passively posed images reported more sexualizing and objectifying statements about themselves than those who had seen the performance-based images. Participants who saw sexualized images were also more likely to describe themselves in terms of beauty or appearance on their worksheets and used more negative descriptors about their looks and feelings toward themselves.

The reverse was also true—those who looked at images of athletes in action self-objectified much less. Significantly, the girls and women who saw the performance-based images wrote more physicality-based statements that described feelings of empowerment based on their bodies as instruments instead of objects. This research brings to light the influence of objectifying media representations of women, including #fitspo, and also the potentially powerful influence of nonobjectifying, athleticism-focused images that can prompt more positive physical self-concepts in viewers. Daniels found that viewing those positive, powerful images did not trigger self-objectification in participants, and may have caused it to subside for some.

More Than a Before

Chasing after fit body ideals is always a bit glamorized in media. The "body transformation" process—by whatever means are being advertised—is made to look hard, but not *that* hard. With the right people showing you how they got there and how you can too (with five payments of $99.99 or by following this exclusive foolproof regimen) and the right combination of dedication, sacrifice, hard work, and motivation, reaching that body ideal oasis looks achievable. And why wouldn't you think you could and should at least *try* to reach it, even if the costs are high? You have been made to feel as if you are lazy and "letting yourself go" if you don't dedicate yourself to pursuing these ideals.

When people decide to transform their bodies, their first step isn't usually to go to the doctor and get a full blood panel and battery of tests to gauge their health *inside* their body. Instead, they step on a scale, wrap a measuring tape around ten different circumferences on their body, and document *how they look* now, before they embark on a new course. They take a "before" photo in their underwear, swimsuit, or workout spandex. Maybe they hide it deep in their photo files, or maybe they post it online to "take accountability for where I'm at and mark the exciting beginning of my fitness journey!"

These photos are often accompanied by a caption about how embarrassing this is and how *I can't believe I've let myself get to this point, but I'm determined to change my life and get my body back!* Sound familiar? Probably. And if it was you who posted it, that's okay. But we want to put this widespread practice in a new light in order to help all of us see more in our health — more than a "before." More than an "after." More than a body to view and evaluate from outside of ourselves.

We know transformation photos are super fun to look at. In their aspirational way, they give us a temporary high of motivation to improve our fitness. But for many people, "improving fitness" really just means "making my body look more appealing." Incredible "after" photos paired with the latest, greatest diet or exercise plan often work as fitspo that encourages people to engage in exercise and eating habits that prioritize altering the looks of their bodies above all else. It might sound harmless, but if you're earnestly seeking to feel positively toward your body and improve your fitness, it isn't.

Our culture's fixation on defining and advertising fitness through before-and-after photos serves salespeople and companies very well, but it doesn't do the rest of us much good in terms of body image or sustained progress toward real health and fitness goals. One of the major reasons why these transformation photos often distract and discourage people from healthy behaviors is that they reinforce the notion that visible results are the only way to illustrate health success. That is, if we don't see results like the "after" photos on the screen, we aren't succeeding at health and fitness.

Pay attention to how you feel when you scroll through "inspirational" images like before-and-after pics posted by people or companies online, or when you look through your own transformation photos. You might run up against Theodore Roosevelt's hard truth: comparison is the thief of joy. Comparing how you look to how pretty much anyone else looks is going to leave you coming up short. Even comparing your current "before" body to your body ten years ago (which may have then also been your "before" body!) doesn't often induce feelings of joy. Have you ever looked back at a photo or video of yourself from your past and wished you still looked like that? Do you remember how at the time you didn't feel great about yourself either? You may have disliked your body then, yet you're convinced that if you had that body *now* you'd be thrilled! And then you're filled with regret, wishing you had just loved yourself back then when you *really* deserved it compared to the "before" body you're working with today.

The reverse is also true: comparing what you looked like in the past when you were heavier or less muscular than you are now rarely induces genuine feelings of joy and gladness. You will start to wonder how you ever "let yourself go," or take an inventory of the things you still need to improve to look better, or compare yourself to someone else's transformation photos and come up short. What if your "after" looks like someone else's supposedly depressing and unfortunate "before"? It happens, and it hurts. Even the most sincere and well-meaning "before" images and captions about starting fresh and really focusing on caring for yourself and changing your life will inevitably disparage others with similar or less-ideal bodies. It is no one's intention to put anyone else down with their transformation photos, but that reality can't be ignored in an objectifying world that ranks and values bodies according to size and shape. Your "before" *will* be someone else's "after." Your "after" *will* be someone else's "before." Sharing these images online guarantees the possibility of hurting people you never intended to hurt, and hurting your future self.

One truth that these very different starting and ending points in transformation photos can reveal is that the maps we are sold to the ideal–body image destinations we desire are faulty. Sometimes the diets, meal plans, workout regimens, superfoods, or miracle products we try do nothing to our weight, size, muscle tone, cellulite, or whatever is supposedly holding us back from reaching that end goal of feeling fit and healthy. Sometimes that goal is nothing but a mirage. It looks like it is within reach— the map shows it is right over the next horizon, and we can see it shimmering in the distance—but no matter how closely you stick to the course, you just can't get there. If you do manage to change the way your body looks, but you don't experience all the joy, confidence, acceptance, love, and fulfillment you thought you would, then it is a mirage. The map is flawed, the course is unreliable, and both the ideal and the path to get there might have been created to enrich someone else's life, not yours.

Before-and-after photos tend to reinforce the assumption that you can measure lots of things about your life based on how your body looks, whether it's your health, happiness, desirability, or self-confidence. **When you learn to see more in yourself and your health, you see that the look of your body does not always correlate with your health or happiness.** It's just not the way our bodies or our lives work.

Many people run marathons; complete triathlons; swim for miles; dance for hours; have balanced eating habits and perfect blood pressure, cholesterol, blood sugar, and resting heart rates and good cardiovascular health — and *still* don't have a body you would ever see in a fitness magazine or even a typical "after" photo. Alternatively, lots of people go to unhealthy extremes like disordered eating, over-exercising, using steroids and unsafe diet pills, and cosmetic surgery to achieve the *look* of health.

Let's not forget that these transformation photos are so easily manipulat*ed* and manipulat*ive*. Check out the hashtag #30secondtransformation on Instagram to see people taking "progress" photos thirty seconds apart to prove how easy it is to simply pose in ways that appear to reflect major weight loss and improvement in muscle tone. Anyone can easily add filters and use photo editing apps to create a truly unreal "after." These images rack up big engagement whether they're real or not.

The reality behind those "after" photos may not always be improved body confidence, self-esteem, mental well-being, or happiness. Yes, some people who post transformation photos are much happier and more body confident in their "after." But many people aren't any happier and don't feel any more positively toward their bodies "after" than "before"—especially if their lives now revolve around restriction, deprivation, monitoring, and obsession with food and exercise.

We probably all know on some level that weight loss or appearance "improvements" don't always equate to life improvement, but the idea that there's a simple formula for success is so alluring. It is comforting to believe that a specific set of strategies to achieve an attractive appearance can lead us to the life we want. If the course and outcomes are predictable and controllable, even if the goal or destination is far off in the distance, we find solace in the belief that, with enough discipline and motivation, we can get there. Do *these* things to get *this* body, and with *this* body, you can have *this* kind of life. We are so often sold this map, with all its evolving variations, as a means for securing romantic relationships, social acceptance, self-esteem, and physical health. But when we really look around at the reality of our world, that map falls apart.

We all know that happy, fulfilling, lasting relationships—whether romantic or otherwise—aren't guaranteed to those who find themselves in ideal-looking bodies. And we know chronic illness, disease, disability, and death do not skip over people who do all the right things and look all the right ways. We know our happiest times don't always come when we look our "best" and our hardest times don't always come when we look our "worst." As much as we want to believe "before" photos always represent depression and lack of self-control while "after" photos always represent perfect discipline, self-love, happiness, acceptance, and endless confidence, these are myths. Extremely common, money-making, hope-generating myths.

From Lindsay: I learned this lesson for myself after I spent a whole summer at age eighteen doing everything I could to lose weight in pursuit of a more appealing "after" body. I isolated myself, walked miles and miles every day, ate tiny portions of food with zero nutrition, and motivated myself with thoughts of how confident, happy, and attractive I would feel when all my friends and new boyfriend came back for school in the fall. Lexie did the same thing, and even though we shared a college apartment bedroom (the last time we ever lived together, praise be!), we were tense and competitive and barely spoke to each other. In that miserable summer, I got down to my lowest weight since middle school. I went home to my parents' house one weekend before fall semester started and tried on some of my old clothes.

On August 17, 2004, I wrote in my journal: "Last night, I tried on my old pants from Christmas of senior year and they are huge beyond belief. I distinctly remember wearing them and feeling pretty good about myself at choir practice, and now I can't imagine ever fitting into them or feeling good. I've gotten more compliments than I can count, and it feels so good even though I don't feel so great about myself. I hope that eventually changes."

I still remember how great I felt less than two years before that journal entry, talking with my friends during choir practice, wearing what I felt was a really cute outfit—a stretchy, maroon three-quarter-sleeve polo shirt and dark bootleg jeans. I even remember how much I weighed, about forty pounds more than when I later wrote that 2004 journal entry. Yet somehow, I felt better in my body then, in those "huge beyond belief" jeans, than I did in my starved, exhausted, *almost* ideal weight "after" body. I was set up for failure all along, and it stung.

That experience, one among many in my life of weight fluctuation and non-correlating happiness and health, reminds me that I am a contradiction to what before-and-after pics often try to claim—and so are you. **You are not a before or an after, whether you love what shows up in the photo or you don't.** Your weight gain and weight loss and muscle gain and muscle loss are just that—weight fluctuations and muscle fluctuations. They are not the full picture of your health, nor of your happiness or fulfillment.

When we can get out of our own heads and stop thinking of ourselves and our health in terms of how we appear to others or compare to other snapshots from our lives, we can better focus on how we actually feel and what our bodies can help us experience and accomplish. It really is possible to reach fitness milestones and accomplish amazing health goals and feel that incredible rush of adrenaline and endorphins without those feats making a visible (or visible enough) difference in our bodies to show up in an ideal "after" photo. Self-objectifying thoughts and behaviors water down and devalue our sacrifices, growth, and strengthening experiences by limiting them to just what we can see. When you are mindful of what health choices mean and feel like in your life, trying to prove or demonstrate that hard work and dedication with a simple photo of your body is doing a disservice to what you

are actually accomplishing. What if instead of thinking of yourself in static, reductive terms of "before" or "after," you thought
of yourself as *in between* those two points: *during*. Any photo you
take of yourself right now is just a "during" shot, captured as you
experience your ever-evolving, ever-learning existence.

Failed by Faulty Goals

As long as your ideas of health are defined by beauty ideals, you
are set up for failure. The sad reality of so much of the profit-driven fitness industry is that by equating *looking* fit with *being*
fit, it actually leads people *away* from better health. You might
turn to unhealthy means to achieve your body goals at any cost,
or, alternatively, become discouraged and turn to a more sedentary lifestyle or binge eating to cope. Both alternatives are damaging, and we have seen and heard countless examples from girls
and women who experienced them.

One young woman who was part of our research shared about
her experience of posing on stage in a "bikini fitness" or "figure
competition." "I have grown up with feelings of low self-worth
regarding my appearance. The hardest time for me I can think of
is last June, when I was in my first fitness bikini competition. I was
fitter and leaner than ever!! However, I still HATED my body!
I knew I was being judged against other girls' bodies by judges
and the other contestants. Most of them looked 'better' than I
did, and I hated that! I worked so hard and achieved so much, yet
I felt more self-conscious than ever! I couldn't have been more

dedicated to my success. Yet, I felt unsuccessful. The day after the competition, I was so exhausted from giving it all I had with 'no' success, I gorged on food. I did that the next day and the next and the next..."

These competitions don't demonstrate cardiovascular fitness, stamina, strength, metabolic health, or any other indicator of physical fitness, just a standardized ideal look that is appraised by a panel of critical judges and an ogling audience. The tales of what happens behind the scenes and in preparation for those leanness-focused events are extreme, and not at all health promoting. No legitimate doctor recommends severe dehydration, malnutrition, laxative and stimulant abuse, and emergency-level exhaustion for anyone's health regimen, but those are often part of achieving the winning competition aesthetic.

Visual appeal is absolutely not the best way to evaluate health. For one thing, the goal of how you want to look can remain out of reach no matter how much you diet or exercise, because your body can't quite conform in the way you hoped. Or, when your body does conform, the result is often nearly impossible to maintain because of the dedication and sacrifice it demands of you. That feeling of failure becomes a major barrier: If you have tried and failed, why keep trying and failing? This barrier to fitness is particularly true for women. One fitness study of both men and women found that the women overwhelmingly believed they had failed at their exercise goals if they didn't lose weight, even if they stuck to their regimens perfectly. Alternatively, many of the men who actually gained weight during the study period still considered themselves to have been successful. The researchers rightfully warned, "It is possible that women's perceived lack of success in weight control when no changes in weight ensue may prompt the adoption of aggressive and possibly harmful weight-loss methods, and exacerbate negative body image and weight preoccupation."

Yep, that's exactly what happens. When women see the goal and reward of exercise as weight loss or a particular physical appearance improvement like flat abs, a round behind, or toned legs, and that doesn't happen as they expected, they think they've failed and are much more likely to give up on exercise altogether or lean into the other end of the spectrum with over-exercising, also known as "exercise bulimia."

That showed up in the ways our study participants defined their own health and fitness goals and whether or not they considered themselves healthy or fit. Multiple responses included feelings of shame or discouragement at not achieving appearance-related results from exercise or positive health choices. One participant described being enrolled in Weight Watchers and doing "P90X" and "Insanity" workouts, yoga, resistance training, and jogging. She hadn't missed a day of working out for three straight months. When asked if she believed she could achieve health and fitness, she said, "Yes, of course. It just takes a lot of determination and hard work. Sometimes it gets discouraging when you don't see the results you want right away, but it's a lifelong battle I think." Her statement regarding "not see[ing] the results you want" becomes noteworthy when put into context with her reasons for pursuing health and fitness, which she stated as: "I look in the mirror and see so much that needs to be improved. I've never been able to look in the mirror and feel satisfied."

Another woman participating in our study expressed similar discouragement at not "seeing" results from her exercise regimen. She wrote that she did think it was possible for her to achieve health and fitness, saying: "A year ago, I ate really healthy and exercised every day. I was able to lose weight, but it was slow going and it kind of went out the window ... I know I'm overweight, like really overweight. I start thinking that I should start exercising, but then I think how ridiculously hard it is to ever see results and then I get frustrated and give up."

These women were doing all the right things to be fit, but their bodies and scales—or mirrors, measuring tapes, or selfies—didn't reflect the physical changes they were taught to expect. They are not alone in being programmed to think that thinner is better, fat is gross, hunger is necessary, and restriction is self-control. When we transgress those rules, come up short in self-comparison with others, or aren't able to maintain the levels of deprivation or thinness we believe we need to, we get discouraged, and we find ways to cope. One response is to binge or compulsively overeat. In a self-protective response to the threat of starvation, our bodies will encourage us to eat and eat and eat. It is a natural and merciful instinct, but too many of us end up in a lifelong cycle—restrict, binge, restrict, binge, restrict, binge—because of the shame we feel about our bodies and our lack of self-control.

At the same time, lots of us cope by *hiding*—quitting our fitness regimen and becoming more sedentary or avoiding social situations, physical activity, or other situations where we might be seen. We might opt out of all physical activity out of lack of energy from food or out of self-consciousness at not looking "gym ready" or being too jiggly. We might sink into depression or live in a constant state of anxiety around food and bodies. At the other extreme, we might exercise for five hours a day just to maintain a smaller size than we are naturally inclined to be. We might spend huge portions of our days meal planning and counting calories or carbs or macros instead of doing something, *anything,* bigger and better and more life giving and health promoting.

We're set up for failure when our body ideals are overpromising on the life improvements they claim to offer, or when they are always just out of reach thanks to the limits of genetics and the false promises of Photoshop and undisclosed surgical intervention. We're set up for failure when our body ideals are impossible to maintain or when they diminish our actual health in the process of changing our aesthetics. When our cellulite doesn't disappear or our love handles don't shrink or our abs or thighs don't tone up, too many of us become discouraged and give up on being physically active and eating a balanced diet. These out of reach body image mirages actually deter us from healthy behaviors like enjoyable exercise and balanced eating, and they become a major barrier to fitness.

One woman told us, "I was always in the overweight category. It made me feel like a failure. Because even when I was working out every day and eating barely 1,000 calories a day and starving, according to my BMI, I was still overweight. I never thought about whether or not it was an accurate assessment of my health.

I realize now that it absolutely was not. It's comforting to me. As long as I can remember, I've been considered 'overweight.' Maybe now I can start thinking of myself as something else."

You can start to see yourself as something else — something more than a body to be looked at — by learning to see more in your health than just your fatness or thinness. When you judge and evaluate yourself by how you appear, you are objectifying yourself. Similarly, when you judge and evaluate your health and fitness by how you appear, you are objectifying your health and fitness. You are doing yourself a huge disservice.

While learning to see ourselves and our health as "something else" other than a size or weight might "comfort the afflicted" in many cases, we understand that this shift in thinking can have a reverse effect and "afflict the comfortable" (to borrow an old quote about journalism from humorist Finley Peter Dunne). Those whose bodies naturally or with minimal effort put them in the category of looking "fit" (in this case, we'll call them the "comfortable") might feel afflicted by this shift away from aesthetic ideals toward other markers of health and fitness. One woman told us, "That actually made me feel bad. I am naturally thin even if I am sedentary . . . Maybe it made me feel bad because I know it's true to a degree — I should be much more active."

Another said, "I was falling into that trap and thinking I was healthier than I am because I am not fat, I have a thin stomach, and I am confident about the way I look in a swimsuit. In fact, I have very little endurance and I am not as fit as I might appear, simply because I don't exercise during the week as much as I should to actually be as fit as I want to be."

It is okay to have your understanding of your own health and fitness be disrupted. If you feel resistant or defensive in response to this suggested shift away from thin ideals, take some time to sit with that discomfort and consider what you're feeling. It is okay to be uncomfortable, frustrated, and resistant to changing the deeply rooted beliefs and hopes about the body you've grown up and grown older with. You might be feeling some cognitive dissonance if this perspective is clashing with the way you've been thinking about your body or your health. This is especially possible if the new perspective feels potentially true and if it asks more of you than your previous view required. You might be experiencing a wave of disruption to your body image that is threatening to push you out of your comfort zone. You get to choose how to respond. Take this disruption to your body image as an opportunity to practice some self-reflection and self-compassion.

No matter your size or shape, your BMI and weight do not define your worth, and they do not define your health, either.

Be More Instrumental

We need to embrace a new paradigm; one that does not stigmatize people for their size, but rather encourages everyone to engage in healthier behaviors for their own intrinsic value . . . Fit and healthy bodies come in all shapes and sizes. And we need to acknowledge that the roads to a fitter and healthier body are wide enough for everyone.
—Glenn A. Gaesser, PhD

So how do we put this knowledge into action? We need to reclaim the reality of what health and fitness mean for each of us, starting with correcting misconceptions and distortions of health and fitness so we can see them as they really are and always were. Your health was *never* really improved by or dependent upon looking a certain way, yet the lie that thinness and good health are inseparable is rampant. Correcting that lie gives us the freedom to define and measure health for ourselves in ways that truly serve us and are truly within reach.

When we've grown up and lived so much of our lives thinking of our bodies and our health from the outside, it takes a big perspective shift to understand ourselves from the inside. This is true for our entire sense of self and how we engage with the world, but especially for our understanding of our own health and fitness. When our bodies are understood and monitored from an inside perspective, we can experience a much-needed paradigm shift in the way we understand health and fitness. We define and summarize this paradigm shift through one simple mantra: *My body is an instrument, not an ornament.* This mantra shifts your outlook from form to function and feeling, from an outsider-focused view to an insider knowledge. **Our bodies are instruments for our own personal use, experience, and benefit—not ornaments to be admired.**

At first, the idea of giving up on achieving weight goals and aesthetic ideals might make you feel like you are giving up on your health or your body. The reality is, letting go of aesthetic goals frees you up to find a new, more effective and empowering way of understanding and experiencing health and fitness for yourself. You can better understand and improve your health and reconnect with your body by focusing on actions over aesthetics, on being an active subject rather than a passive object to be looked at. Don't decide what you want to weigh or how you want to look—decide how you want to *feel*, what you want to *do*, and what you want to *experience* along the way.

Fitness over Fatness

This instrument-not-ornament shift isn't some nonsolution to make people feel good about being in bad health—this is research-backed health promotion that puts the focus on achievable, controllable behaviors and outcomes rather than arbitrary and unattainable weight goals and aesthetics. Glenn A. Gaesser, an exercise science researcher at Arizona State University, summarized some of his findings in a university publication, stating: "Our current focus on weight loss has been an abject failure. During the past 40 years or so, Americans have collectively undergone more than two billion weight-loss attempts, mostly by dieting. Yet during this same time obesity prevalence has tripled. Not only has dieting not worked, it may have contributed to the increased prevalence of obesity."

In the 2010 book *Health at Every Size: The Surprising Truth About Your Weight*, Lindo Bacon, PhD, writes, "The only way to solve the weight problem is to stop making weight a problem—to stop judging ourselves and others by our size. *Weight is not an effective measure of attractiveness, moral character, or health.*

The real enemy is weight stigma, for it is the stigmatization and fear of fat that causes the damage and deflects attention from true threats to our health and well-being." The Health at Every Size movement aims to "advance social justice, create an inclusive and respective community, and support people of all sizes in finding compassionate ways to take care of themselves." The HAES approach emphasizes how social and economic issues play a more prominent role in our health than the individual behaviors that receive so much of the focus. This has proved to be a radical concept in a culture that has been so immersed in aesthetic-focused definitions of health. A quick Google search of "Health at Every Size" reveals years of backlash against the movement and debate about whether it is irresponsible to suggest that people considered "overweight" or "obese" by the medical system could also be metabolically, cardiovascularly healthy at their current sizes —or even just whether it would be okay for larger people, and all of us, to focus on other health indicators than their body size.

Despite the slowly evolving mind-sets of people in a fatphobic society, there is lots of agreement in research that healthy behaviors—including but not limited to regular exercise, avoiding harmful substances like cigarettes, and eating a balanced diet—are more important factors in a person's health than their body size—and that social conditions trump all. Research continues to show that a person's level of physical activity is a better indicator of their health and fitness than their BMI or weight—and an even greater determining factor is their zip code. Researchers are encouraging people to think of these larger social factors (like where and how you grew up, your job and income, and how wealth and resources are distributed among communities) as "root causes of health" because of how significantly they impact a person's health outcomes. Much rhetoric about health places the burden of achieving good health squarely on individuals without regard for all the larger contributors to health disparities that can't be fixed with lifestyle changes.

When looking at individual behaviors, multiple studies have found that cardiorespiratory fitness is a better predictor of a person's risk for disease and death than their weight or BMI—even for people who are considered "obese." One groundbreaking 2007 study showed that people who are overweight and active may be healthier than those who are thin and sedentary.

"When we look at these mortality rates in fat people who are fit, we see that the harmful effect of fat just disappears," researcher Steven Blair told the *Guardian* in March 2010. He was describing the 2007 study he coauthored, which measured 2,600 older adults' fitness and weight, and then followed them to compare all of their chronic disease and mortality rates. "If we look at individuals who are obese and just moderately fit—we're not talking about marathon runners here—their death rate during the next decade is half that of the normal-weight people who are unfit. So it's a huge effect."

These findings turn the ideas most people have about health on their heads. They challenge every mental image we have about who can be fit and who can't, who is healthy and who isn't. Many of the judgments we pass on ourselves and others because of weight and appearance are unfounded and simply wrong.

Focusing on fitness rather than fatness is well proved to de-

crease risks of numerous diseases and disorders, including diabetes, multiple forms of cancer, hypertension, and other causes
of death. Doctors who care to explore a person's health beyond
their weight know this is true. When people with serious health
issues like type 2 diabetes, cardiovascular disease, and high blood
pressure start a meaningful exercise program, their health problems often disappear or greatly improve—regardless of whether
or not they remain classified as "overweight" or "obese."

The overwhelming takeaway from these findings is that rather
than relying on your BMI or weight to indicate your health, a
better strategy is to take a critical look at and acknowledge the
systemic factors outside of your control that may be impact-
ing your health, and then focus on practicing healthy behaviors
within your control. One long-term study of almost 12,000 people of all sizes pinpointed four important lifestyle habits for living a healthier, longer life: eating five or more servings of fruits
or vegetables daily, not smoking, limiting alcohol consumption,
and exercising at least twelve times per month. In the study, these
habits were associated with a significant decrease in mortality
regardless of BMI—in other words, the people who practiced
those four healthy habits lived longer, regardless of whether they
were categorized as "normal weight" or "obese."

Food and Intuition

Not smoking and not drinking too much are pretty straightforward and widely accepted practices for good health, but lots of

people might be surprised to see the inclusion of eating fruits and vegetables as opposed to restricting other food groups. In our diet-obsessed culture, many so-called health coaches would tell you to eat fewer calories or carbohydrates and cut down your sugar intake by eating vegetables instead of starchy snacks or fruit in lieu of dessert. The focus is on what you should subtract rather than what you should add. However, we know this restriction mentality not only doesn't work for long, but also backfires, leading most people to feel deprived and then "slip up" and go wild on off-limits foods, or even teaching them to associate fruits and veggies with punishment or dissatisfaction.

Professor Traci Mann (whom we mentioned earlier for her psychological research on dieting) said her lab has taken a non-diet approach to promoting this particular healthy behavior, focusing on making vegetables more appealing rather than using them as a means to calorie restriction. In a brief for the APA, she said, "Our most successful strategy aims to minimize the 'competition' vegetables get from less healthy and more-liked foods." She described serving vegetables as the first course of a meal rather than serving them as one portion alongside everything else, where they might get passed over. "This strategy was successful when used with adults who were watching videos in a lab setting," she wrote, "and it led to dramatic increases in vegetable consumption among elementary school children who were served vegetables before they entered the cafeteria for lunch."

Making it easier to improve health habits is a good strategy. However, that doesn't remove the shame and stigma many have internalized around which foods are "good" and "bad." Some restrictive diets ban fruits and some vegetables (say goodbye to carrots and potatoes!) in order to avoid even natural sources of sugar, all in service to weight loss, with no regard to health or nutrition. We have been fed so much pseudoscientific diet culture misinformation that food has become a minefield for lots of people. What we "should" and "shouldn't" eat varies from week to week and "expert" to "expert." This drives people into endless cycles of harmful restricting and bingeing, which messes with our metabolic systems, our hormones, our health, and our lives.

To combat this, dietitians have been working for decades to help people create healthier relationships with food. The pioneers in this space include Evelyn Tribole and Elyse Resch, registered dietitians and the authors of *Intuitive Eating: An Anti-Diet Revolutionary Approach,* which aims to help readers "make peace with food, free yourself from chronic dieting forever, and rediscover the pleasure of eating." Their methods help people reconnect with the internal cues for hunger and fullness that we all naturally followed as toddlers — eating when you're hungry and stopping when you're full — as well as teach people to trust their bodies, rather than rely on externally prescribed approaches to food through diets.

Christy Harrison, registered dietitian and the author of *Anti-Diet: Reclaim Your Time, Money, Well-Being, and Happiness Through Intuitive Eating,* calls our culture's dieting obsession (aka diet culture) "the life thief." She writes, "Dieting is against your best interests. It puts you at war with yourself and takes your energy away from fighting so many more important battles. It makes you doubt yourself and feel like you can't trust your own instincts. It gaslights you into thinking that you're the 'failure' because you 'couldn't stick to' the diet du jour. Because you had the audacity to get hungry, to need nourishment and pleasure. To need the things we all need. That's abuse, and yet The Life Thief is an expert in getting us to perpetuate it on ourselves, again and again and again."

The solution to getting off the diet roller coaster and learning to trust your own body is to take a more mindful approach to food and body image. Both of the aforementioned books are fantastic resources for learning to eat intuitively. *Making the locus of control our own senses and intuitions rather than profit-driven diets is a powerful way to gain a more balanced relationship with food and to reconnect with our own bodies.* For people whose ideas about living a healthy lifestyle are dominated by restrictive diets and exercising for weight loss or maintenance, unlearning those ideas and learning new ones takes lots of conscious and self-compassionate effort.

It is important to be aware of how kids are dealing with the food and diet talk that is likely surrounding them, as well. If you want to avoid pulling your kids into the waters of objectification to struggle alongside you, you have to start by fixing your own faulty beliefs and habits. Throw out your diet books. Unfollow thinness-focused accounts and influencers. Ditch your bathroom scale. Eat that slice of birthday cake with everyone else. Don't moralize food as "good" or "bad," but instead talk about the ways it makes you feel, the variety of flavors and colors that are important to have, and the vitamins and nutrients that help your mind and body thrive.

What should you do if your child starts restricting food or expressing an interest in dieting? Let them know that many people and companies in this world try to convince people, especially girls and women, that they should shrink and take up less space, but it's a mean lie. This lie is intended to get people to spend money and time worrying about their bodies instead of living and leading and serving and taking up space doing good in the world—and, too often, it works. Talk to them about how our bodies need and want food for lots of reasons, including for fuel and for enjoyment, and that by paying attention to how they feel when they eat, they can take better care of their bodies and trust that their bodies will lead them toward choices that are good for them and that have nothing to do with their body size or shape. Let them know strict diets hurt our bodies by confusing them about what to do with the food we eat—in fact, sometimes they prompt our bodies to store more of its energy than we really need, because our bodies think we might be starving and are trying to keep us alive.

Personalizing Your Health

Unfortunately, for both adults and kids, developing or maintaining a more holistic, non-aesthetic view of our health is hard in our world, whether because of rampant objectification or simply tradition. Kids in school are sent home with their BMIs listed on their report cards. A routine and unquestioned aspect of almost any medical checkup is being weighed, often with your weight and BMI reported to you and discussed at the visit. The desire to avoid even knowing these numbers is an understandable aspect of shedding your dependence on them. It's much easier to not obsess about your weight if you don't have that number in your mind. What many people don't recognize is that this automatic weigh-in at the doctor's office is not mandatory for the majority of appointments, and getting out of it is often as simple as requesting to skip it. If the provider insists it is relevant or medically necessary for this particular visit, you can always ask to turn around so you don't see the number and request that they don't report it to you or discuss it with you unless medically necessary. For those who are able, this is a great step toward advocating for yourself at the doctor's office—a place where too many people feel stigmatized and intimidated because their health complaints are so often attributed to their weight without regard to anything else.

From Lexie: For my second pregnancy, I decided I didn't want to be weighed at every monthly or twice-monthly prenatal appointment. I decided this for three reasons: first, because that number and the associated BMI posted at the top of my personal medical records are fraught with meaning that our culture assigns it, and I have worked hard to get over my allegiance to those numbers; second, because other factors like blood pressure and blood sugar are more indicative of my health; and third, because I want to advocate for others who are too afraid to go to the doctor because of having to be weighed and judged for that weight. Specifically requesting not to be weighed and explaining my reasons why was my way of reminding my health care team that I was a person first, and my health cannot and should not be defined by my weight.

When I asked not to be weighed and explained my reasoning, the midwife at my university hospital absolutely agreed with me and honored my request. She told me that at her practice, they wanted to ensure pregnant patients are gaining weight—not losing it—and that's why they measure weight at each appointment. We agreed I would be weighed once per trimester and that I not be told my weight or have it discussed unless they felt it necessary for my health. Not every medical provider will be so kind, and not everyone is in a position to ask for this accommodation. But the more of us who work up the courage to try, the better. I went through my entire pregnancy being weighed exactly once, and was never weighed again during postpartum checkups.

My health care providers and I were able to determine my health status, without getting on a scale, by all the other indicators measured during pregnancy: regular blood tests, urine tests, taking my temperature, blood pressure screenings, etc. Having successfully opted out of weigh-ins throughout my pregnancy gave me the confidence to continue to opt out since then, and I have not been weighed at any of my other appointments that used to take my weight, like my regular skin checks at the dermatologist. Knowing I didn't have to be weighed and congratulated or side-eyed at any of my appointments was a huge relief, and significantly decreased my anxiety around my changing body.

If you're looking for a way to get a better grasp on your health status than what a "before" picture or scale displays, consider checking in with your doctor or other trusted health care professional. Be open that you are working to avoid focusing on weight, size, and any other appearance-oriented goals. Ask for help to get greater insights into your health, including your blood pressure, resting heart rate, blood sugar levels, cholesterol, risk factors for illness or disease, and even just feedback on your lifestyle and habits or how you're feeling about your overall wellness. Your provider can help you understand what your ideal internal measures of health might be, and what you can adjust to achieve those goals. If they can't help, or they aren't willing to skip the weight discussion, it is time to look for a new health care provider, if possible.

As you are working to reclaim your own personal understanding of your health and fitness, keep in mind that they are highly individual pursuits that are relative for anyone. What is considered healthy and fit for one person might be substantially different from what is considered healthy and fit for another person. Health and fitness are not entirely within our control for a million reasons, including disease and illness and socioeconomic barriers like limited access to good health care and nutritious food (just consider how expensive it is to buy produce!), limited physical ability, and little free time for exercise, among many other factors. It is also a dynamic spectrum, not a simple stopping point or destination where you get a mark of "healthy" or "not healthy."

Some people might hope to stave off illness, disease, pain, or even death through being hypervigilant about health and fitness, but none of those things is truly within our control. So much of the health and "wellness" industry preys on people's very real and warranted fears of debilitating illness and disease, but there are no surefire ways to ensure you never get sick or lose the ability to enjoy the function of your body. Even if you do your very best to appreciate and understand your body as an instrument instead of an ornament, that doesn't mean your instrument will work as you would like it to.

Instruments aren't invincible. They fail us, they hurt, and they can feel like a burden, but they are still instruments—not ornaments. This is a truth that can be adapted to wherever you are at the moment, whether you're dealing with a chronic illness, an injury, a disability, or any physical limitation. Are your lungs allowing you to breathe? Is your heart pumping your blood? Are you able to see, smell, hear, or touch? Can you communicate your thoughts and feelings? Can you write, create art or music, or enjoy hobbies and talents? All of these actions are made possible by having an instrumental, not purely decorative, body. Don't get stuck in stereotypes or ideals of what you think an instrument needs to do or be.

The fact that each of us has a body—regardless of our appearance, health status, fitness level, or ability—means that we innately have access to physical power in some form. This is an inherent power that we ignore and forget when we remain focused on how we appear from the outside. That power and the way we access it is going to vary for every single person because we have wide-spanning differences that greatly affect the use of our bodies and our experiences within our own bodies. Not all people will be able to improve their health and fitness or enjoy the use of their bodies for physical activity, but all people can benefit from developing an appreciation for the function of their bodies—however limited—rather than simply their aesthetic form.

Using Your Body as an Instrument

Setting your sights on new health and fitness goals means taking your sights *off* the looks of your body. To put this new instrumental perspective into practice, you need to do two things: 1) let go of your objectified ideas of health and fitness, and 2) learn to define health and fitness in ways that are achievable and sustainable in your own life. Fortunately, the first one increases the likelihood of the second pretty dramatically. When, in our doctoral studies and through our online body image resilience course, we have asked women to define health and fitness for themselves, about 40 percent of participants tended to answer in terms that included a distinct appearance focus. When we asked how capable they felt about achieving health and fitness (aka their self-efficacy to achieve health), about 25 percent of our study participants expressed serious doubts about their ability to do so. That was not at all surprising, since as long as it was being defined by often unattainable appearance ideals, fitness would be out of reach for most women. Those who felt furthest from the ideals felt the least capable of becoming fit, often after many failed attempts to lose weight that solidified their feelings of hopelessness.

Those participants then spent a few weeks delving into our online course, which included a health information "intervention" covering the ideas we've shared in this chapter. They learned how inaccurate simple measurements like weight and BMI are for understanding their own health and fitness, and about the research that shows physical activity is a better indicator of a person's health and fitness than BMI, weight, size, or any other external measurement. They reflected on the examples of people in their own lives who might look like the aesthetic definition of "fit," but may not have lifestyles or health reports that demonstrate good health or fitness, as well as the many people who don't represent traditional "fit" body ideals but achieve fitness feats and experience great health and strength.

After learning to see more in their own definitions of health, almost all of our study participants who initially felt health was out of reach showed a significant increase in their self-efficacy to achieve health and fitness. In other words, once they shifted their thinking about health and fitness to be based on how they feel and what they do rather than how they look, they felt much more confident and in control of their health and fitness outcomes. Some even went from feeling hopeless about their fitness to recognizing that they may *already* be healthy and fit, once they got the focus off of their weight or appearance.

One woman said, "That actually made me feel a lot better. I've always been a pretty active person, and I love that even though I'm not the skinniest girl in town I can be healthy." Another said, "I just started training for a 5K with my friend. Already it feels way more satisfying to track if I can run for a longer period of time than if my weight is down. I'm really excited about it!"

Others shared their motivations for improving or maintaining their health that didn't rely on their weight or appearance. One said, "Both of my parents have had health problems starting in their 40s and I don't want that. They lived average lifestyles, minimal exercise and poor eating, and I want more for my life than that. I want to be able to provide opportunities for my kids that I never had and that means pushing myself more physically and mentally to be strong, active, and healthy."

Another said, "Overall, I think it means being able to use your body in the ways you desire rather than being limited by it. For example, being able to participate in any activities or take care of any problems or get anywhere you need to be or do anything you want to do without worrying that your health will prevent you from doing so."

Focusing on how you feel and what you can do will get you much further than simply focusing on decreasing fatness. Physical activity, when approached with the right mind-set and expectations, can be a powerful tool for improving your body image. It can help you reunite with yourself as you experience the power and privilege of your body as your own. Your new mind-set relies on your internal, first-person perspective on your body and your goals. One of the greatest benefits of engaging with your body in this way is that when you are able to experience a powerful, instrumental sense of self, you are less prone to self-objectify. It requires effort and energy to experience your body through movement, but by doing so, you can decrease your tendency to body monitor and self-objectify while also increasing your stamina, strength, speed, and capability as you experience your life in a whole new way.

This mental shift can also help break down some of the barriers that might have been holding you back from being active in the first place. In response to the question "What has prevented you from engaging in healthy behaviors or activities?" one woman told us, "My body shame. I would skip out on social outings or even group sports because I didn't want to be the ugliest/fattest one there. I would avoid going to the gym because I was too self-conscious." Her response echoes the many other women quoted in chapter 3 who were ruled by self-objectification, body monitoring their very lives away.

Researchers have found one of the most significant barriers to exercise for people categorized as "obese" is their body image perception, with "feeling too fat to exercise" showing up as one of the most common hurdles, particularly for women. A study based on data from the 2002 National Physical Activity and Weight Loss Survey found that body size satisfaction had a significant effect on whether a person performed regular physical activity, regardless of the individual's actual weight. That is, those who felt okay about their body size — no matter their size — were more likely to engage in physical activity regularly than those who felt crappy.

On the flip side, getting involved in any kind of athletics or enjoyable physical activity is a practical way to boost your body image because it can help shift your perspective toward what you are doing and feeling instead of how you look or what you weigh. It might take some work to get out of your comfort zone — and starting a new form of physical activity or moving from sedentary to active might be a body image disruption in itself — but it can have a huge impact. Countless women have told us how much sports and exercise have improved not only their fitness but also their self-perceptions by helping them avoid self-objectification. In many cases, they left behind sports as teens or college students and remember their experiences with proud nostalgia.

One woman who participated in our research said, "In junior high, I spent all my time wrapped up in athletics. It's what I loved, and I excelled at it. I was a softball player. A catcher. A short setter in volleyball. I was proud of my physical abilities, believing I could do anything I put my mind to. I LOVE exercise. I love the way it makes me feel. It's because I want to be able to feel strong, powerful, and confident. There is a sense of accomplishment when a certain speed or mileage is accomplished—a joy that cannot adequately be described."

When women start working toward action-oriented fitness goals or start participating in a sport after previously measuring their fitness according to their appearance, they often feel a sense of empowerment and recharged confidence in their physical abilities.

One woman in our studies said, "I have started biking and I am super excited by the way my body has responded. I have quadrupled my distance within 3 weeks, even after having the flu last week." Another said, "I feel happier when I exercise regularly and I love the feeling of improving—of being able to run faster than I could before, or dance all through Zumba more easily than I could when I first started going." Those little victories are easily overlooked when all we're measuring is what shows up on the scale or in the fit of our jeans.

One woman shared with us her example of initially sinking into shame while trying to lose weight. She said, "After I had a baby, I began starving myself." Too many women's stories end there. But her story didn't, because the pain of starving herself served as a wake-up call—a disruption to her body image. She said, "I realized I needed help. I began reading literature about body image, including [your blog], and I set a goal to run a 10K. I have been focusing on being healthy enough to train for that. Even though it is still hard for me to weigh more than I want to, I am focused on health and strength now. I had to weigh more to be strong enough to run, which is what I love to do. I also find that it's important to focus on what I can offer the world, which is a lot more than a number on a scale or a dress size. I have a lot to offer!"

How do you avoid the pitfalls of setting fitness expectations that keep you focused on your body as an ornament rather than an instrument? The difference can be pretty difficult to tease out if you've been immersed in objectified thinking about your health. Ask yourself: Is my goal asking me to measure my fatness or my fitness? If it's measuring fatness, your goal destination will be visual and literally, physically, measurable—pounds, inches, dress sizes, muscle definition or tone, BMI score. If it's measuring fitness, your goal will be invisible and based on what you want to feel, what you want to do and experience, or what you want your lab test results to reveal. Your goal will look like climbing X flights of stairs without being winded, walking or running a certain distance each week, doing X repetitions of bicep curls with X pounds by X date, getting your heart rate in a certain range for

X minutes every day, decreasing your blood pressure or choles-terol, leveling out your blood sugar, etc.

A key to this mental shift is going into exercise activities or fitness regimens with *no* assumptions about what effect they will have on weight, size, shape, cellulite, or body proportions. It can be difficult to shake the hope that our efforts to be active will shape our bodies in particular ways, but getting your mind off of those body ideal oases will pay off in the future as you pursue reachable, empowering goals instead of mirages.

Test out what it feels like to focus internally rather than how exercise might impact you externally. You can do this by find-ing any type of movement you enjoy and doing it mindfully and consciously while taking inventory of what you like (and don't like) about it. Which muscles are being engaged? What is your breathing like? How do you feel in the process? If and when your attention goes to how you appear, push it back to what you are doing or experiencing. If you catch your mind worrying how your arms look while they jiggle each time you move them, shift it to focusing on how it feels to move your arms in that way. What does the air feel like on your skin? What do you appreciate about this moment, how you're feeling, or what you're doing? Do you feel any changes in your mood or energy level throughout this movement?

Additionally, make sure you take time to turn your attention outward, away from your body. Enjoyable physical activity pro-vides a great opportunity to get into a flow state, in which your attention is fully on the task at hand and nowhere near your ap-pearance. For women who are constantly being dragged down and distracted by the wet jeans of self-objectification, escaping that burden even for a few moments can be truly transformative. When have you felt that escape and relief from hyper-self-awareness?

Autumn Whitefield-Madrano, author of *Face Value: The Hidden Ways Beauty Shapes Women's Lives,* wrote about seeing female athletes in a flow state, free from self-objectification.

> When you're in the act of wanting something badly enough, there isn't room for self-consciousness. How you look, your stance, your hair, your makeup, whether you appear pretty, your sex appeal: all of these things that coalesce in my brain, and maybe yours, to form a hum so low and so constant that I take it as a state of being —and when you want, they disappear. When you want, the want goes to the fore. Then you can take a back seat . . . Certainly there are plenty of times in every woman's life when how she looks isn't at the fore of her mind, but it's rare to have proof—visual, irrefutable proof—that at that moment, she is absolutely not thinking about how she looks. To watch female athletes is to watch women not give a sh** when they look ugly.

Choosing Instrumental vs. Ornamental Activities

Seeing other women who are using their bodies as instruments instead of ornaments can inspire us to engage in a less self-conscious way with our bodies. But in a world where the objectification of women is the norm, not all sports and exercise activities are created equal. Ask yourself, "In this activity or sport, are women's bodies used or viewed as something instrumental or ornamental, or both?" In general, competitive teams or individual sports or activities in which the players' performance is evaluated purely on what they do—make a basket, score a goal, hit a home run, earn a point, jump the highest, or run a distance—don't emphasize the players' appearance. No scoring system evaluates their aesthetic appeal. No points are withdrawn for not looking ideal. Basketball, soccer, softball, football, tennis, swimming, running, track and field, lacrosse, rowing, water polo, and so many more fit into this category.

Alternatively, some sports and activities *do* place a value on aesthetics—cheerleading, dance, ice skating, and gymnastics are all examples. These are still great for improving fitness, but they can nevertheless have negative effects on body image and promote self-objectification since they can heighten pressure to be thin and heavily made-up, to align with highly specific beauty ideals. That doesn't mean they are evil or must be avoided at all costs. It means that if you participate in these activities, or want to, you should be aware, cautious, and proactive about mitigating their possible negative effects. We know this not simply by watching how women are scored and judged, but also because of what girls and women report from their own experience.

One woman told us, "I grew up dancing and cheerleading. These are two sports where your body image gets seriously distorted. I remember when I started at a new cheerleading club in 8th grade and my mom told me that we should make some changes if I wanted to look like the other girls … I've always been very aware of my own body and other people's bodies. I don't know if this is because of media, being involved in dance and cheerleading when I was young, or what. I'm just very aware."

In aesthetically oriented activities, self-objectification is built into the sport. A constant awareness of how your body appears and how closely it resembles highly specific (and always thin) ideals is baked into anyone's participation and success. Some coaches, judges, parents, and teachers make the pressure worse; fortunately, some try to alleviate it.

Author, dancer, and instructor Amanda Trusty wrote a great piece for the *Huffington Post* in which she describes the instructions she heard over twenty-four years of ballet training that revolved around sucking in her stomach, squeezing her bottom, and other commands intended to keep her focused on looking perfect. She wrote, "I realize now where all my insecurities started. They started in first position at age seven at the barre. And now here I am, 20 years later, catching myself doing the same things to my own 7-year-old students. Oh, but I refuse … How can I tell my ballerinas to suck it in and tuck it under, knowing how much that shaped my childhood?"

She spent the next several weeks reimagining the usual directions given to girls in dance in ways that don't stigmatize anyone's body size or place a premium on thinness. In place of the common instruction "tuck the booty under, don't let it stick out when you plié," she substituted the request "send your tailfeather down instead of out." She says she asks her girls to envision that they have a "beautiful tailfeather" connected to their tailbones. Instead of telling them to hide or squeeze their bottoms, she asks them to dip their tailfeather into a pool of water below them. She says, "The tailfeather concept keeps their pliés perfectly aligned without them ever thinking about how big their booty is at all."

Trusty's innovative approach is a great example for all parents, coaches, and instructors who have a responsibility to be aware of the effects of their language on girls and young women. Regardless of the norms and traditions in any given sport or activity, we all need to consider how the instructions and reminders we give girls might be reinforcing the same objectifying messages that negatively impacted each of us earlier in life.

Be on the lookout for how body-conscious workout gear might impact you, too. Researchers Ivanka Prichard and Marika Tiggemann found that women in fitness centers who wore tight and fitted exercise clothing placed greater emphasis on their appearance attributes and engaged in more habitual body monitoring than women who wore looser clothing like T-shirts and sweats or joggers. Researcher Peter Strelan and his colleagues found that the attention focused on women's bodies in fitness centers—for example, through mirrors surrounding them in gym classes—leads women to self-objectify more. Less body-baring uniforms and workout gear can help alleviate body consciousness and promote better performance. They also put female and male athletes on a more equal playing field because the same sport shouldn't require significantly different uniforms. Running or going to the gym shouldn't come with wildly different pressures and expectations of how body conscious women's and men's gear should be.

If you have felt "too fat to exercise" or too self-conscious in your workout clothes or athletic uniform and have held yourself back from physical activity, try to take your mind off how you look. Avoid working out in front of mirrors, or if you need a mirror to check your form, check your form as needed and then look away. Alternatively, look yourself directly in the eye and consciously reconnect with who you are and what you are experiencing as you use your body as an instrument, not an ornament. Experiment with different clothing choices. Skin-tight, pastel-colored activewear might be cute and Instagrammable, but if it keeps you thinking about how you look, try something else. Opt for baggier clothing or more coverage and see if it helps. Where possible, talk to your instructors and coaches about wanting to get your focus off of your appearance and on to your performance by wearing more comfortable attire, even an alternate uniform or one you can modify to fit your needs. Professional basketball players wear compression tights, spandex, and T-shirts under their standard uniforms all the time. Do whatever you need to do to feel your best and perform your best.

A Better Kind of Before and After

Undoing the effects of objectification on your health is a challenge, but it is possible. You absolutely can reframe your perspective about your body to take on a more instrumental focus, even after a lifetime of judging it for its ornamental value. We have seen that in our own lives and in our own research. Consider this a new and improved kind of "before and after" health and fitness transformation. Here are three real-life examples from our study participants, given before and after three weeks of them learning to see more and be more.

Before: "I don't really like my body. I can't remember a day that I woke up and was glad to be in the body I'm in. My thoughts are often about how I could or should lose weight, and I feel very guilty if I eat food that I know will cause me to gain weight. I'm grateful for my body but I wish it looked different, mostly just that I was thinner."

After: "I am grateful for my body, especially because I am very healthy compared to a lot of ailing people in the world. I have all my limbs, my organs function properly, I don't experience pain every day, etc."

Before: "I feel very self-conscious. It's never looked how I want it to. There is cellulite, scars, veins . . . things I try hard to keep hidden. I always think, 'Why can't I look like her?'"

After: "I still feel like it's a work in progress. It's imperfect, but it's mine, and I am working on making myself feel good about it. I think our bodies are amazing, really. They are capable of so much when/if we push them to do so. When I focus on that I feel much better about my body. I am so impressed with my body that I was able to complete a 12-mile obstacle course five months after having a C-section!"

Before: "My body can be frustratingly flawed in looks and performance. It aches and gets tired, and certainly is not very pretty to look at (especially without clothes). I don't like the 'muffin top,' flat chest, and cellulite on my legs . . . I try to stay pretty content with my body if I don't see all the other images or a particularly unflattering picture of myself."

After: "I feel much more satisfied with it. I know that my body has the energy and strength to do fun and active things with my family . . . Honestly, I don't think at any size I will think my body looks amazing, so I am going to try to stop defining my satisfaction with it by how I look. I feel tough and strong and like I can keep up with any task given to me."

Gaining greater understanding of your health requires a broader look at all the factors that contribute to how you experience your body—both in terms of the systemic inequities that affect your family and community's health outcomes, as well as the personal ways you've been taught to objectify your health. When you can see more in your health than the numbers and appearance ideals you might have been trained to focus on, your body can become an instrument for your own use and experience rather than an ornament to be admired, fixed, and judged. With that shift in perspective, you can have greater access to your own physical power that comes through experiencing your body from the inside, not the outside.

6

A Resilient Reunion

- What sources have you turned to for help to learn how to feel better about your body?
- What kinds of self-help strategies for do-it-yourself body image improvement have you heard about or tried?
- Which ones have helped, and which ones didn't?

See More in Your Self-Help

> When women lose themselves, the world loses its way. We do not need more selfless women. What we need right now is more women who have detoxed themselves so completely from the world's expectations that they are full of nothing but themselves. What we need are women who are full of themselves. A woman who is full of herself knows and trusts herself enough to say and do what must be done. She lets the rest burn.
> —Glennon Doyle, *Untamed*

In the waters of objectification—where our body images are being toppled by waves, pulled by currents, dragged down by sopping clothes, and led astray by faulty maps—how do we sur-

vive? How do we help ourselves toward better body image solutions? Negative body image is a complex problem with complex
answers, but the most popular strategies to address it over the
past couple of decades haven't succeeded at pulling us from the
depths of despair and distraction. Many have even reinforced the
objectification of women's bodies. As long as our efforts to promote positive body image are focused on feeling positively about
how we look, we are still being objectified.

While the popularity of body positivity and increasing body
diversity in popular media show that our culture has certainly
made progress toward acceptance and inclusivity of more than
one ideal body type, we haven't made similar improvements in
the way girls and women feel about their own bodies. Fifteen
or so years after the launch of widespread efforts to promote
positive body image through expanding ideas of how "beautiful"
looks, girls and women seem to be suffering as much or more
than ever under the burden of body shame. When news agency
Agence-France Presse asked psychoanalyst Susie Orbach about
the difference between women's body image issues in 2018 and
more than forty years ago, when she wrote the best-selling book
Fat Is a Feminist Issue, she said, "It's much, much worse than we
ever envisioned. There are all kinds of industries both creating
and feeding off these insecurities ... If you just dropped in on
any conversation, the amount of mental space that people take
up with what they're eating, what they're not eating, their yoga
routine, is expressive of the level of distress in our society."

The root of the problem that popular strategies haven't been
able to crack is in the way our culture understands body image

in general. We have grown accustomed to thinking of body image as a visual, viewable version of ourselves that can be entirely understood and perceived from the outside. ***Your body image is not the literal image of how your body appears, or even your feelings about how it appears. It is your feelings about your body — the body you live inside, grew up with, and experience life through.*** Your body image can be perceived only from the inside and understood only from within. It's the difference between the question "How do you feel about your body?" and "How do you feel about the way your body looks?" In order to better understand how and why our self-help efforts might have fallen short in the past, let's deconstruct some of the most recognizable body image improvement messages of the past couple of decades. Once you learn to see more in your body image self-help, you can learn to help yourself more effectively.

The Business of Body Image

"You're more beautiful than you think."

The Unilever-owned body products company Dove became well known starting in 2004 for its viral "Real Beauty" ad campaigns, which featured women in their underwear in a wider range of sizes than usual, and then had another viral hit with its "Real Beauty Sketches" ad campaign in 2013. After having an artist sketch women in the way others described them (traditionally beautiful) as well as in the ways they described themselves (less beautiful), the video ended with the tagline "You're more beautiful than you think." Dove's next viral campaign, which debuted at the Sundance Film Festival in 2014, encouraged us to "redefine beauty one photo at a time" by taking selfies and recognizing our beauty. We discussed the flaw of this message earlier in this book (on page 116).

Dove isn't the only company or well-meaning organization or campaign taking aim at body shame through this general strategy. "You're more beautiful than you think" is equivalent to messages like "You are beautiful just the way you are" or "Your flaws make you beautiful." Of course, we all want girls and women to feel beautiful, especially after a lifetime of feeling subpar in comparison to unreal ideals. This approach is an understandable response to decades of one-dimensional beauty ideals and cohesive messaging about which bodies and faces are acceptable and worthy of love. But even when it's billed as something we *are* rather than something we're *not*, this constant emphasis on beauty signals and resignals its cultural importance for girls and women.

When you look closely, the maps to achieving beauty, fitness, and improved body image often look strikingly similar. The courses and strategies to get there might be different, but the destination is the same: feel beautiful. And even if you think you're embarking on a journey of self-help and improved body confidence, it can be just as elusive as more mainstream beauty ideals. Changing currents of beauty standards, disruptive waves of shame that throw us off course, and differences in ability, genetics, and a million other factors will prevent most of us from fitting even expanded beauty ideals and feeling great about our looks consistently.

We believe women are suffering not only because of the ways *beauty* is being *defined;* we are suffering because we are being *defined by beauty.* We are burdened with the task of *looking* beautiful and *feeling* beautiful (to others as well as to ourselves) because we live in a world that defines our value in terms of our physical appeal to others and defines our body image in terms of our physical appeal to ourselves. Being viewed as objects is the real root of our problem, not which beauty ideals are in vogue for female objects.

Body image improvement campaigns and efforts that focus on improving the way girls and women feel about the ways their bodies *look* keep them stranded in the waters of objectification, at the mercy of cultural currents in comfort-zone life rafts that are constantly at risk of deflating, flipping, crashing, and sinking. These strategies provide only temporary relief and the illusion of making "progress" toward better body image by countering our body shame with messaging about how beautiful we *really* are.

While it might not be an effective strategy for major cultural change, the "you're more beautiful than you think" messaging has been very effective financially. Dove's two ads based on the "Real Beauty" sketches received more than 35 million views within their first couple of weeks on YouTube. The company's sales jumped from $2.5 billion to $4 billion after starting its Campaign for Real Beauty. Dove's messaging and inclusion of "real women" (*their words, not ours*) in advertising has endeared the company to women who are hungry for expanded ideas of beauty.

Further, since this strategy to improve body image maintains beauty as the hallmark of our value, the company is *also* able to capitalize on women's insecurity and body fixation. They can say "real is beautiful," but they have still made millions on products that promise to fix distinctly female beauty problems that are the definition of "real," including "skin-firming" cellulite-minimizing cream and "even tone" "underarm makeover" deodorant for "softer, more beautiful" armpits. They have very successfully marketed the same old beauty products to women—all while invoking the language and imagery of activism. This is commodified body positivity. It isn't evil, but it is profitable. More on that in a bit.

"EveryBODY is beautiful."

In the last several years, online activism known as #bodypositivity or #bopo has boomed, challenging ideas of what it looks like to have a "good" body and encouraging more people to believe "everyBODY is beautiful." Body positivity is all about appreciating the look of the body you have, as well as appreciating the diversity of bodies in our world. This is hugely important to acknowledge in a world that historically has only appreciated a few ways to have a body.

This is a mainstream offshoot of activism that started in the fat acceptance movement, with body positivity springing from the truth that many women's bodies have been excluded and erased from mainstream media or depicted as abnormal and shameful. It's perfectly natural for women to want to see themselves as beautiful and acceptable and want themselves to be seen as beautiful and acceptable by others. They want others with similarly invisible shapes and features to see the bodies they never saw when they needed to see them. So, among other things, the most prominent #bopo stars share and celebrate bikini selfies and lingerie photo shoots that often include body types that have been marginalized or made to seem shameful or inferior in mainstream media. They are taking their power back from mainstream media that almost never features diverse women in positive, happy ways by representing themselves on their own terms.

The body positivity movement offers a safer alternative to chasing unrealistic or unsustainable body ideals. Instead of trying to reach an impossible destination in order to feel confident, body positivity suggests you can achieve the hoped-for effect by reenvisioning yourself as already being there. Body positivity truly is a life preserver for many people who are in the depths of body shame, gasping for air in the sea of objectification. Its messages of comfort and appreciation for bodies that don't conform to the narrow ideals celebrated in our culture can feel liberating. When you feel crappy about your body and you first see someone who looks like you unapologetically embracing her body with no hints of embarrassment for her size or appearance, it can be incredibly validating. People can find comfort in seeing their own looks being celebrated online and normalizing their own body types.

This strategy for improving body image by sharing and validating images of a broader range of women's bodies is extremely popular and certainly represents a much-needed life preserver for many, but its effectiveness has its limits. We think of body positivity like a life preserver because it provides temporary reprieve from the negative effects of body shame for some people, but no one intends to just hang on to a life preserver forever, even if it is extremely helpful in a time of need. Unfortunately, even with the reminders to love and accept your body as it looks right now, you are still stranded in the waters of objectification. Expanded ideas of which bodies are considered "beautiful" or acceptable are still keeping a focus on how those bodies look. It keeps individuals focused on valuing their own bodies for how they look, which keeps us bogged down with the burden of self-objectification even if we like how we look.

Body positivity life preservers can still get swept away from us by crashing waves of body image disruptions that overwhelm us with shame. Maintaining a grip on positivity about your body is often impossible in the midst of an environment where we value beauty over everything and where "beauty" is defined in such limiting ways by so many people and industries around you. What happens when you (inevitably) lose sight of your beauty in the face of so many contradictory messages about what it means to be beautiful? And what happens when your own body is simply too different from the others represented within the body positivity community to really find comfort or safety there?

What happens when the most popular, mainstream, celebrated #bopo activists reflect all the same mainstream beauty ideals except with slightly larger thighs or rounder bellies? Traditionally beautiful white girls with perfect skin and able-bodied women with hourglass figures on the lower end of the plus-size range may easily find solace and solidarity in the body positivity movement—while women of color, those with disabilities, those who don't conform to stereotypical feminine looks, those beyond the acceptable size and shape range, and those who don't have enough money for the best brands and styling might still feel invisible, ignored, or looked down upon. Questions at the intersections of race, class, and ability have rightly become a topic of concern in the body positivity sphere. ***All too often, well-meaning people and companies end up reinventing the same limiting ideals that benefit some and marginalize others, just in a slightly expanded range of sizes.***

This life preserver can keep your head above water when needed, but it doesn't produce the lasting, radical transformation we need. When we focus our body image improvement efforts on embracing the many looks of women's bodies, it can be hard to tell what is empowering and what is simply re-creating the same objectifying conditions we were already drowning in. In these conditions, how do we differentiate between stereotypical sexually objectifying images of women's bodies—which are intended to arouse (mostly male) audiences and demean and diminish women—and #bopo images that are intended to be subversive and empowering for female viewers?

For women who are publicly posting body-centric photos online as a sign of embracing their supposedly flawed bodies, where is the magic line that determines when a post turns from emulating standard objectifying images that often *hurt and minimize* women to displaying progressive body positivity that *helps* women? Is it automatically empowering and progressive if she's over a certain weight or size? Or if she doesn't like the way she looks, but she posts it anyway? Or if her stretch marks or cellulite are visible? Or if she's basically an ideal size, but she's hunched over to create a belly roll?

Sure, the *intention* behind a body positivity post is very different from the intention behind a standard objectifying image of a sexualized female body meant to be consumed by others. But if you take away the inspirational caption, it is more of the same: female bodies being bared, shared, compared, evaluated, and ogled. **Validating and appreciating the diversity of bodies that exist, while inclusive and helpful on the one hand, still centers the appearance of women's bodies as their most important feature.** This approach still depends on women being awarded arbitrary points for what their bodies look like, just with expanded guidelines for what counts as worthy of displaying or consuming.

"All bodies are bikini bodies."

The popularity of this appearance-centered brand of body positivity has redefined how a woman is expected to demonstrate her body confidence. It can be summarized with one viral and trusty slogan: "All bodies are bikini bodies!" And if that is true, then it must be proved! *Pics or it didn't happen!* Wearing a bikini and posting the proof on Instagram has become the gold standard for demonstrating body confidence. Yes, of course *every body is a bikini body* if that's what you really want to wear, but why have so many of us bought into the idea that wearing a bikini means you love your body *and* that loving your body means you must wear a bikini?

We argue it's the same reason so many of us struggle with low self-esteem and negative body image in the first place: the core belief that your appearance defines your worth. When our looks are the *most* important thing about us and when body confidence gets minimized to simply embracing the *looks* of our bodies, it makes sense that bikinis—the most revealing of all publicly acceptable attire—take on otherworldly power in our lives. We call this bikini tyranny. Why tyranny? Because no item of clothing can or should have that kind of power over us—for good or evil. For so many years, bikinis have been put on a pedestal reserved for only the "hottest" among us. In recent years, with much-needed body positivity activism, women have worked to topple that pedestal in order to help people of all sizes feel comfortable enough to wear one.

Sure, there are lots of great reasons to wear a bikini, if that's what you want. It might make going to the bathroom easier during a day at the pool. It might prevent the uncomfortable groin and shoulder strangulation of a one-piece that is too short in the torso. It might allow for a much nicer tan. It might look awesome. It might feel like liberation from "modest is hottest" or "don't be a stumbling block to men" ideas you grew up with. But it might also spark constant monitoring and tugging and adjustment if you're moving around much, let alone trying to play or swim. It might expose too much sensitive skin to the sun (*not again, melanoma*) and sand and saltwater and hot chairs. It might be impractical and uncomfortable and trigger you to constantly think about your appearance—in fact, that last piece is extremely likely, whether you love the way you look in a bikini, hate it, or feel somewhere in between.

You might wear a bikini because you love the way it looks or feels. You might even wear it to push back against beliefs about your body being sinful or being someone else's property. *Awesome.* We love seeing body diversity in media *and* at the pool or beach. Everyone deserves to swim, and to be comfortable while doing so. But pretty much no one asks men to prove their confidence by posting Speedo pics on Instagram. (Well, straight men, that is. Gay men face similarly heightened body pressures as women do online and off, with much of the origin of both traceable to the sexualized male gaze of who is doing the looking, evaluating, and consuming—regardless of the gender of the person being consumed. Scholar Mitchell Wood expanded Laura Mulvey's 1975 idea of the "male gaze" to include the "gay male gaze." He writes, "Increasing the complexity of this objectification, gay men are both the subject and the executors of objectification of other males.")

In a world of objectification, revealing more of our bodies online might feel like the truest path to liberation and empowerment, and it might seem like bikini pics are the best way to demonstrate self-love and confidence. But we disagree. We want to let swimsuits be just that: items of clothing to wear in the water. Not badges of honor or tests of courage or proof of pride. Our swimsuits prove nothing about our body images and they shouldn't have to. They're just swimsuits.

Commodified Body Positivity

So many of these swimsuit-oriented, beauty-focused strategies for positive body image have been embraced by the mainstream not because they are overwhelmingly effective, but because they are profitable. Grassroots, activism-oriented #bodypositivity has been co-opted by companies and individuals who are simply capitalizing on a trend to seek profits—something we call *commodified* body positivity. This profit-driven knockoff looks a lot like something truly groundbreaking for women, but it's most often a simple rebranding of a product, service, or company, and these companies often continue to marginalize and objectify women and profit from their insecurity.

It might look like progress for women, but it always costs, and that cost often benefits people who don't care the slightest bit about how you feel about your body, and who maybe even hope you'll feel like crap because they also happen to sell some other stuff to fix your flaws. Cough, *Unilever.* Cough, *Weight Watchers.* Cough, *Sports Illustrated* swimsuit issue. Cough, *too many to name.* Yeah, yeah, yeah, that's capitalism. **We know! But audiences and consumers are manipulated to feel like progress for marginalized people is being made when it's usually only profits from marginalized people being made.**

Commodified body positivity convinces progressive and conservative people alike to cheer when notoriously sexist and objectifying outlets like the *Sports Illustrated* swimsuit issue include models who are a few sizes larger than their typical centerfolds or feature beautiful young Olympic gymnasts who are more muscular than their male audiences and advertisers have generally preferred. Those women may still be down on all fours, mostly nude, or totally nude but painted, breasts in hands, with lips pouted and parted, pulling down bikini bottoms, backs arched —*you know, all the expected positions for gals in the world's most popular sports magazine*—and yet this is branded as body positivity and is then applauded as progress for women.

Let's be clear that this magazine is *only* in the business of making millions off of this particular issue and its advertisers by providing sexual stimulation for onlookers and #bodygoals for women. We can't let the *Sports Illustrated* swimsuit issue or any other historically sexist medium be our barometer for women's advancement. Expanding the boundaries for which bodies qualify to be objectified for profit does not translate into actual empowerment for women, but it certainly translates into mega-sales for media outlets and their advertisers.

We will always advocate for more diverse representations of all women in media, but we'll know progress is happening when those same women aren't required to take off their clothes in order to be included. We need substantial, regular roles and representation for women of all shapes, sizes, colors, and ability levels that do not revolve around how they look, their weight-loss "journeys," or how sexually appealing they can be. We want inclusion and representation, not equal-opportunity objectification.

The same sneaky commodification of body positivity shows up throughout social media as companies and influencers figure out that #bopo not only looks and feels like activism for social good, but it is also lucrative. The most-liked pics of women on Instagram are the body-baring ones — no matter how those bodies look. Bodies get the likes and the views.

When a lifestyle blogger posts a casual swimsuit pic of herself in front of a cool brick wall — laughing and flipping her hair, captioned with an explanation of how she doesn't love how her thighs look in this photo but it's more important not to be embarrassed and to inspire other women; or when an Instagrammer smiles at the camera in her underwear, hunched just slightly to reveal skin folds as a middle finger to beauty standards; or when a new mom with a big following posts pics of her not-quite-as-flat (but almost!) abs while claiming bravery about embracing her new postpartum body on her journey to "get her body back" . . . they know they'll get maximum likes, comments, and engagement. They, and most people, might even call those posts #inspo, #goals, or even "empowering."

But are they? If you strip away the inspirational caption and good intentions from so many of those #bodypositive posts, are they really just capitalizing on a feel-good social justice trend as a marketing strategy to sell whatever sponsored product is tagged in the photo, or to increase engagement for their next #ad? Or is it just another pic of a woman's undressed body for viewers to compare, ogle, and double-tap? If the "body positive" images and messages we are celebrating (and sharing and liking and retweeting and buying) are indistinguishable from the sexism and objectification that have always been used to *devalue* and *disempower* women, then they might not be all that revolutionary.

What originated as a feminist and political tool to push against oppressive ideals and stigmatization of marginalized people in the form of fat acceptance has largely become a watered-down version of body politics to push products, not progress. And when body positivity becomes a sales strategy, we have to look at what is being sold. Who is the *consumer* and what is being *consumed?* Sometimes the products for sale alongside images of undressed women of all shapes and sizes and #bodypositive statements are goods that cater to and fill gaps in the market for women of all shapes and sizes — underwear and swimsuits, for example. *Awesome and yes, please.* But sometimes the products for sale are goods that capitalize on the insecurities of women of all shapes and sizes and their desire to be worthy of consumption. And sometimes the products for sale are simply undressed women's bodies in all shapes and sizes, presented for appraisal, validation, and consumption.

Body positivity has been appropriated as another way to turn women into consumers and women's bodies into the objects being consumed, only this time a wider variety of bodies qualify for consumption. This isn't a matter of serving the greater good; it's simply a matter of *selling* goods. If it didn't sell more goods and gain more views and more likes, then the sellers and influencers would find a new strategy. But it sells. Because women eagerly consume other women's bodies in media in an attempt to validate their own worthiness to be consumed. Audiences eagerly participate in these disguised marketing campaigns by liking and retweeting and sharing what appear to be empowering images and messages, while those messages effectively serve to enrich the seller—whether the seller believes a word of their #bopo message or not.

And all along, the problem intended to be solved by body positivity activism—*negative body image*—remains firmly intact. We monitor our bodies, consciously and unconsciously working to adjust our appearances to be most appealing to onlookers. Self-objectification is happening in the minds of the body positive influencers and the millions of onlookers scrolling through the influencers in their feeds, comparing their parts and aspiring for whatever they don't have. That's a prison. Objectification hurts us. It minimizes us, it distracts us, it drains us. It always has. Only now, under the guise of commodified #bopo, we've been duped into thinking our body-centric system of value is also our path to empowerment.

"Look better, feel better."

"I did it so I could feel better about my body. I did it so I could feel more like a woman. I did it so my clothes would fit better. I did it for *me*." This is the onscreen monologue of a national TV commercial for breast augmentation, spoken by a white, thin, blonde woman who looks like the prettiest mom in a rich neighborhood. Gone are the days of daytime commercials with a male doctor explaining the life-changing benefits of enlarging some parts of female bodies and shrinking others. Now, it's by women, for women. It's what I want, not what men want me to have.

Women and teen girls are seeking cosmetic procedures such as breast enhancements, liposuction, abdominoplasty (aka "tummy tucks"), and rhinoplasty (aka "nose jobs") in record numbers. This is a testament to the effectiveness of advertising messages and consistent media content with the sometimes blatant and often subliminal promise of "look better, feel better." Those two are inseparably intertwined in so much of advertising geared toward women, as if surgery is really self-help. As if our looks really have the power to determine our feelings. This message might not sound like a traditional positive body image slogan, but it functions in the same way. Cosmetic surgery is promoted by advertisers and satisfied customers alike as a tool to increase women's confidence and improve their body image, all under the premise of being "for me" and to "feel better."

However, if you are considering an operation like breast implants to feel better about your body, you should know that it isn't the surefire solution it might seem to be. For years, studies have explored links between breast implants and increased rates of suicide in women. Researchers have been seeking to understand whether undergoing breast implant surgery increases a woman's risk of suicide or whether mental health issues increase the likelihood for women to undergo breast implant surgery. In a 2016 in-depth analysis of all fifty-two peer-reviewed studies published on breast implants and suicide, researchers Diana Zuckerman, Caitlin Kennedy, and Mishka Terplan concluded: "Scientific evidence suggests that breast implants may have risks to mental health. Although suicide among women with implants is below 1 percent in every study, the rates ranging from 0.24 percent to

0.68 percent are significantly higher statistically and clinically than rates for comparable women without implants. Rigorous research is needed to better understand the consistent association between implants and suicide, and to determine how to decrease those risks for the 300,000 US women who undergo implant surgery annually."

They recommended systematic measurement and long-term tracking of implant patients as well as mental health screening before implant surgery to identify women who may be vulnerable to depression or suicide. Importantly, the researchers noted: "The high suicide rate clearly suggests that breast implant surgery should not be considered a solution for low self-esteem or depression, as is sometimes suggested in advertisements and was policy in some European public hospitals and for British and Australian military women." Cosmetic surgeons have contacted us with this same acknowledgment after recognizing that their patients are seeking surgical procedures as therapy, or as sincere attempts to feel better about themselves, to decrease depression, or to improve romantic relationships, and they have seen firsthand that their work does not live up to that hope or hype.

More than 300,000 women and teenage girls underwent breast implant surgeries in 2018—a threefold increase from 1997. We don't believe this boom in breast augmentations is being driven by overwhelming body image success stories—it is being driven by women's shame about their natural breasts. Breasts that look nothing like the ones consistently featured in mainstream media and the vast majority of pornography because they aren't perfectly round or "perky" or evenly sized and they change after pregnancy and breastfeeding and weight gain and loss and illness and age.

What does it really mean when a woman who undergoes cosmetic procedures says, "I did it for me"? Unless the person saying this is into recreational surgery, then what this statement might really mean is: "I did it to look better." When women elect to undergo cosmetic procedures on the premise that it's "for me," they're almost always speaking from a place of self-objectification, or viewing their bodies from an outsider's perspective. They're saying they like how they look more when they're seeing their own reflections or wearing a swimsuit, and when others are looking at them. In turn, they're saying they'll *feel* better because they will think they *look* better. (Note that we're not talking about surgery for mastectomy reconstruction, gender confirmation, or to address pain or health complications.)

The reality of why some women might feel better after cosmetic surgery is that they receive more acceptance and validation from others (and themselves) for their more ideal-looking bodies. If cultural ideals didn't teach us all that certain boobs are better than others, millions of girls and women wouldn't be getting medically unnecessary objects implanted in their chests. If we take "look better" and "get more validation from others" out of the equation, what's really in it "for me" at the end of the day is: spending thousands of dollars; losing significant time in surgery, recovery, and follow-up exams; possibly losing sensation in your breasts and other operated-on areas; and risking your health, including through common complications, increased chances of cancer as well as *decreased* chances of detecting cancer, the little-studied but massive phenomenon of "breast implant illness," and more.

Instead of admitting and acknowledging that cosmetic procedures—whether breast augmentations or butt lifts or Botox—are profit-driven pursuits that overwhelmingly prey on women's body shame, the cosmetic surgery industry convinces women that elective procedures are self-care, self-improvement, and a quick fix for body image woes. ***But self-care that is truly caring takes care of your whole self, not just your visible self. Self-objectification is not self-care.***

Moving Beyond Beauty

In a culture that values women for their bodies more than anything else, we learn to seek our self-worth through our bodies. We learn to search for scraps of what sometimes feels like empowerment in the form of validation and acceptance of our bodies. It's understandable. Those scraps of faux power can be a satisfying reward in this system, and it isn't difficult to look around and see examples of women reaping the rewards of looking desirable. The reason we call this faux power is that it is based on others' whims and preferences. The rewards for fitting beauty ideals or being deemed desirable are attainable *until they aren't.* He changes his mind. She finds a better option. A new "look" is in. You get older. Your appearance changes. You become sick or injured. You get pregnant. You run out of money.

When your empowerment is based on others' physical appraisal of you, it can be taken away as freely as it was given. It is fleeting and fickle. Lasting, meaningful empowerment doesn't come from believing that your body looks acceptable or even having your body be accepted by others. While that is a good feeling and can certainly provide satisfaction, there is much greater power to be found outside the confines of woman-as-object. Empowerment is a broadly defined concept, but we're using it to describe a personal, self-determined sense of capability, confidence, and self-worth. When a woman is empowered, she is in control of her own sense of self rather than having it defined or determined by others. Her self-worth won't falter when someone tells her it should. Our profit-driven culture convinces us that our bodies are where our ultimate power lies, but this is a lie. We all fail in a system that values only our bodies at the expense of our humanity. Objectification is not some natural part of what it means to be a woman. The only way to fight it, and the corresponding internalized self-objectification, is to call it out. To see more in it, shine a light on it, and understand how harmful it is to call it "empowerment" and "self-help."

If you are interested in improving your body image and self-worth in a culture that values you as a body first and a human second, then you have to look critically at your own ideas of empowerment and self-improvement first. It is up to each of us to learn and recognize the difference between well-intentioned but short-sighted solutions, those that sell us ideals or products while perpetuating our body fixation, and real, positive body image solutions that help us improve our relationships with our bodies, not just our visual perceptions of them.

The big problem with all of these messages—"you're more beautiful than you think," "look better, feel better," "everyBODY is beautiful," and "all bodies are bikini bodies"—is that even if they are perfectly effective at convincing us they're true, we're still stuck in a rut. Even if we are successfully convinced that we're more beautiful than we imagined and already have a bikini body, the constant monitoring of our lovely appearance is still a distraction and a detriment to our lives. The well-documented harms of self-objectification remain whether we *like* our looks or not—and the likelihood is still that most women don't like their looks, or like only certain parts of themselves temporarily.

So what is the alternative? Instead of trying to map a course to a destination of "feel beautiful," where do we want to end up? What should be the end goal? We suggest the possibility of a brand-new beach destination marked with a big red *X* on your body image map: More Than a Body. There, we understand that positive body image isn't believing your body *looks* good, it is knowing your body *is* good, regardless of how it looks. This destination is reachable, and reaching it is transformative.

We want more people to experience that transformation, and since we started running our nonprofit and sharing our work online and through social media in 2009, we have watched and participated with great interest as body image has become a major buzzword and part of the cultural conversation. We also became aware of the shortcomings of body positivity, especially commodified body positivity. Starting around 2015, the difference between what we were personally doing to promote positive body image and what was being *called* positive body image in the mainstream was undeniably stark. It was increasingly hard to see so many people's and companies' online followings explode only after they started sharing heavily body-centric content in the name of body positivity (and often in name only, while still selling weight-loss miracles and flaw-fixing solutions). This pattern so clearly matched what had *always* been valued about women as long as our images have been documented—bodies first, humanity second.

We know that lots of companies and individuals adopted this strategy to make sure girls and women could see the reality and variety that exists in our bodies. They worked from the understanding that women whose bodies historically haven't qualified to be seen in media are being marginalized. *And they are.* But we wanted, and still want, to push for a deeper understanding that *all* women are being marginalized by the very fact of being seen as bodies first and foremost by others and by ourselves.

This distance between what we understood from our research and what was being championed online had been clear to us for a while, but it felt too fraught to publicly acknowledge it because we were deeply involved with so many of the other activists and Instagrammers trying to provide body image inspiration and resources. Offering a critique of any of their tactics and the enthusiastically embraced body positive messaging of mainstream brands felt terrifying, even if the sole intention behind it was to help the girls and women we all care about. In January 2016, we made our first blog and Instagram post about this specific issue, describing it as the "clashing camps in body positivity." We made an image that said, "The first group is fighting for women to be valued as more than bodies to view. The second group is fighting for more women's bodies to be viewed as valuable. We're in the first group. Which side are you on?"

In the caption, we wrote:

This new post is hard to share on IG, where the #body-positivity world thrives with the help of people we love. This comes from a place of compassion and long years of researching body image, so please consider our thoughts. Because our culture teaches that women's bodies and faces determine our worth, and that only certain rare bodies and faces are worthy of anything good, people who want empowerment are stuck in two conflicting groups. The first group seeks empowerment by calling out and fighting objectification — the system that defines women's value in terms of their physical appeal. In this first group, there is no room for lingerie photo shoots or nearly nude selfies, no matter how different the bodies on display might look from media ideals.

The second group springs from the truth that many women's bodies have been erased or made to seem abnormal and shameful. These women want to *see* themselves as beautiful and they want themselves to *be seen* as *beautiful. So, among other things, they share and celebrate nearly nude selfies and lingerie photos featuring marginalized bodies to fight shame. We understand why.*

We must fight body shame, but we need to fight it at its source: the idea that the appearance of our bodies is the most important thing about us. When we try to alleviate shame around certain body types, we're only fighting a symptom of the problem, not the cause. The problem is the fact that women's *bodies* are valued more than women themselves, not the fact that only *certain women's* bodies are being valued. These two groups aren't enemies, but they're fighting different opponents. We in the first group firmly believe the opponent is objectification — the system that defines our value in terms of physical appeal. The opponent is *not* mainstream beauty ideals. Beauty ideals suck, and they're as unattainable as ever. They'll always be here, but it's objectification that holds them in power. Rather than reinventing what beauty looks like, why not push against the whole idea that beauty is of utmost importance? We align with the first group, and we want to be clear about why.

We were right to be nervous to post that, but it was something we could not keep avoiding. If we had written this post today, we wouldn't have approached the issue in such a divisive manner. It's not an either/or situation. Developing body image resilience is a process, and for lots of people, it can begin with body positivity and expanding our definitions of what is considered beautiful and sexy. We were frustrated with the lack of progress beyond all the "I am beautiful and you are too" posts and hoped people would see the difference between that approach and ours of acknowledging the ongoing harms of being viewed and treated as objects. We were met with *lots* of support and a ton of confusion and anger. We were blocked by one of the most popular body positivity activists who had previously been a supporter, and unfollowed by several more, while others grappled with the ideas we presented and wrote about the paradigm shift in their own posts, blogs, and feminist websites. The pushback felt intense, but hundreds of people who were genuinely invested in promoting positive body image really engaged with our message, sharing questions, comments, and their own insights. We watched as our words popped up in others' posts, both positively and negatively, and are grateful that over time, we have been able to see ripples of that shift take place throughout social media in the ways people depict and discuss what it means to develop positive body image.

We were not the first or only people to challenge the ways body image activism sometimes furthers the objectification of women, but it is possible we were the first from within those spaces to say it publicly in those spaces. We are grateful to see the many activists, influencers, and social media users who have moved forward with an awareness of whether they want to focus on only "fighting for more women's bodies to be viewed as valuable" or move toward "fighting for women to be valued as more than bodies to view."

Body Image Transformation

While the meaning of *positive body image* has been twisted over time to signify "loving the way you look," we have continued to push for a more accurate understanding of the term rather than giving it a whole new name. Thus, our whole "not just believing your body *looks* good, but knowing it *is* good" message. In early 2016, following our controversial post, activists began to use the term "body neutrality" as a new way to describe positive body image that isn't about just appearance. ***Body neutrality is the next generation of body image progress — a state of accepting and respecting your body as it is, prioritizing how you feel and what you do*, *rather than how you look*.** Body neutrality builds off what you already gained from body positivity so you keep that helpful life preserver, but it is even more helpful because it also provides respite from self-objectification.

Some people make their way to body neutrality after finding only limited or temporary relief through practicing body positivity. Being immersed in objectification makes it really difficult to hang on to feelings of being beautiful, "flaws and all," while countless sources are mocking, degrading, and convincing you to fix those "flaws." Some people, no matter how hard they try and how many #bopo accounts they follow, can't convince themselves that they are beautiful, and others balk at the idea of prizing beauty at all. The next step forward is finding a nonappearance-focused way to value your body, like body neutrality, and letting that shift in perspective free you up to engage with your body and your life in a new way.

Without being dragged down by the constant burden of self-objectification and the mental task list it enforces, you will find that having a positive body image is achievable and life is more enjoyable. Learning to live your life and understand your relationship to your body outside of evaluating its appearance is liberating. However, accepting your body how it is now does not come naturally for people who have grown up in constant pursuit of the "feel beautiful" oasis. Veering off that course might feel like a cop-out or like you're neglecting yourself, but that is not true. You are simply working toward seeing a bigger, better, three-dimensional map of your life's possibilities rather than the limited, faulty, profit-driven ones you've been offered before. That's not you neglecting your beauty or attractiveness; that is you prioritizing and embracing your best interests.

Maybe you don't have to bob along in the dangerous sea of objectification, forever chasing body goals that disappear like mirages when you try to reach them. By developing your skills for body image resilience and letting those constant waves of disruption propel you in a new direction, you are headed somewhere you didn't think possible. You begin to see land on the horizon.

You are navigating away from a flimsy sense of self-confidence and empowerment that is inseparable from your feelings about your looks. This shift is connecting you with the privilege of living in and through your own body, rather than privileging anyone else's perspective of you. Your empowerment can no longer be handed out to you by validating comments, attention, and engagement and stolen away when the attention wanes. Your empowerment is self-determined, emanating from inside of you, and can never be taken from you. Your answer to that baseline question of "How do you feel about your body?" is being reimagined from inside of you rather than given to you by someone observing you. Your body image is becoming *yours* for the first time. You are putting yourself first, merging your self-objectifying perspective with your own inside perspective, and realizing you are a human being, not just a human being looked at. It's time for a reunion.

Be More Than a Body

> I wasn't unnatural after all; the cultural attitude that taught me so was the real abomination. My body, I realized, was an opportunity. It was political. It moved the world just by existing. What a gift.
> —Lindy West, *Shrill*

The Reunion

In all your years of seeking confidence, acceptance, love, and contentment through all the methods available to you in the waters of objectification, you've probably come up short. You are not alone. There is no shortage of smart, dynamic, successful, high-achieving, forward-thinking, loved, and loving women who have every reason to feel at peace with themselves, yet still feel discouraged and disappointed with their bodies. They *know* they should get over their fixation on losing weight, toning up, slowing down signs of aging, and all the other sexist standards they would tell others to ignore, but they just can't. ***Achieving peace with our bodies through positive body image is the final frontier for too many women — the last and most stubborn barrier to our own confidence, fulfillment, power, and self-actualization.***

Outside forces in your life, like ever-shifting currents of beauty trends and body ideals, have played too large of a role in how you relate to and think about your body. You have been battered by waves of disruption to your body image that have overwhelmed you and left you frantically coping until the danger and discomfort passed. Your comfort-zone life raft has become even less comfortable as your attempts to cling to it through hiding and fixing your body have failed you. When the body ideal destinations you sought all turned out to be mirages, you might have become increasingly directionless and discouraged with yourself — upset at your inadequacy and inability to reach the goals that seem so reachable for others. But now you know about a new destination, More Than a Body Beach, which you can see in the distance.

The only way to get there is to leave behind your comfort-zone life raft — either through a wave of body image disruption that will inevitably push you out, or by choosing your own wave and diving into it. Instead of dealing with your shame and discomfort in the same old ways, you can choose to rise with resilience, letting that wave of disruption propel you in a new direction. You kick off your wet jeans of self-objectification and swim toward the glimmer of land you recognize on the horizon. On the distant beach, you see a figure waving her arms as you approach. She waves with excitement and motions you toward her. As you get closer and the water gets more shallow, she reaches out her arms to help you find your footing upon the sturdy ground you haven't felt beneath your feet in years.

You know her. She is your whole, complex, dynamic, human self, right where she has always been since your identity split and you learned to feel at home in the waters of objectification through your own self-objectification. She is your inner child from the memories and pictures you love from your past, all grown up. The same body you were born in and grew up in and experienced every second of life in. All the bad, all the good, all the pain and joy and highs and lows. She puts her arm around you, welcoming you home to yourself after your long venture to see more and be more. You sit with the sure knowledge that your body *is* good, and you deeply understand that your body is only a fraction of your identity. You have learned so much about yourself in the sea, which makes this reunion all the more powerful. You are home, grounded in the truth that your experiences and pain and responses make you more of who the world needs you to be, not less. You are no longer doubled as the seer and the seen, the consumer and the consumed, the human being and the human being looked at.

To be "more than a body" is to be whole, to be at one with who you are and always were. It is a reunion. It is self-actualization. It is the highest form of self-love and self-compassion in action because you are embracing yourself, regardless of how you appear. You are embracing and finding deep meaning and purpose in what you and your body have been through, and what you will go through in the future. You will no longer blame your body for what you've experienced or the expectations it hasn't met. You won't be divided against your body again. You are your own best and most loyal ally, accepting that pain will come, expectations may or may not be met, others will approve or disapprove, and none of that will turn your body from an instrument into an ornament.

Instead, the pain you experience is an opportunity to reconnect with yourself, to feel yourself slip away, and to know how you can return again, more resilient and whole. Regardless of where you are starting right now, you have the opportunity to step into the brave revolution of rising with body image resilience. This is the capacity and skill set we all need to survive the waters of objectification and reconnect with the sense of self we started with as carefree kids.

When you know (and know how to remember) that you are more than a body, you will find that your sense of self, empowerment, and life possibilities are expanding. You will find out that the path to fulfillment and achieving your personal potential is bigger and better than simply forcing your body to fit a perfect mold.

That knowledge is both liberating and overwhelming because it means finding confidence, happiness, good health, love, and acceptance is messier and less linear than expected. None of those things are guaranteed based on how you control your appearance, despite what every weight-loss or cosmetic-surgery ad suggests, simply because of the nature of being human. However, disconnecting your hopes and dreams from your dream body also expands your own power to reach them. It puts some of the control back in your hands for how you find balance, peace, and fulfillment through the ways you live your life and respond to your disruptions — none of which are dependent on fitting specific ideals that may or may not be realistic.

You will lose the feeling of control you get managing your anxieties by choosing to hide or fix your body to avoid or prepare for a big presentation or social event. You will lose the sociality of participating in conversations about others' weight gain or loss, or the community of participating in the latest diet trend or weight-loss bet and connecting with others about your progress or meal plans, and the bonding of complaining about your love handles with friends or family. You will lose out on some of the fleeting validation that comes from your own beauty work, like weight-loss compliments that have always motivated you to continue dieting, or the self-satisfaction that comes with feeling like you are better-looking (and maybe *better* — period) than someone else who isn't quite as attractive as you. You will also lose your imaginary vision of your future self whose body looks *just different enough* from your present reality that she is magically confident, worthy of love, successful, and happy.

In place of those losses, you will gain so much more.

That job, leadership opportunity, promotion, presentation, or other career-related goal you've been pushing down the road until you make some changes to your appearance? You can have the confidence to try for it now, carrying yourself with greater self-assurance about who you are and what you can contribute to any organization or situation, knowing your capability and confidence aren't tied to your looks. Regardless of what happens, you will be able to interpret the positives and negatives of the situation through a clearer and more compassionate viewpoint that doesn't place blame or credit squarely on your body.

That outdoor activity, sport, game, workout class, or other physical fitness experience you thought looked fun, but your self-consciousness has held you back? You can give it a chance now. You might gain a new hobby or habit that puts you in a better mood, improves your stamina and cardiovascular health, levels your blood sugar, helps you relieve stress, connects you with new friends, and helps you understand your body as an instrument, not an ornament.

The unhappy, emotionally abusive, or otherwise toxic relationship you've been staying in for fear that no one else could possibly be attracted to you? You can walk away and find out what it is like to be respected and accepted by yourself first. Letting go of a partner who tries to keep your self-esteem low so you don't believe you are deserving of anything or anyone better is the best thing you can do for your love life. When you lose that burden, you gain the possibility of finding a healthier relationship with someone who has your best interests at heart, but this time you'll go in with the understanding that you are already whole without a partner. You don't need anyone to complete you.

The physical intimacy you have avoided or missed out on

or faked your way through or felt detached and self-conscious during? You can find greater connection with your partner and increased pleasure and enjoyment as soon as you stop imagining how you appear to them rather than being fully engaged. Learning to let go of self-objectification gives you an entirely new and improved way to enjoy intimacy.

The hard-earned dollars you spend every month on your beauty routine, from hair removal, styling, coloring, and maintenance, to your daily skin care and makeup regimen, your mani-pedis, Botox and fillers, fashion, and everything in between? Add it up. That money could still be yours. Keep it for yourself or use it for something more exciting or fulfilling to benefit yourself or others who need it. For extra motivation, compare it to what almost any man in your life spends every month to maintain or improve his looks. Even more, consider the "pink tax" you have likely been paying (a more expensive price tag for women's products compared to the same products for men, because they are made extra special, just for you, and being special comes with a price!).

The waves of jealousy or competitiveness you sometimes feel when seeing someone else is looking extra great or getting attention you wish you had? They can go away, or at least lessen. When you reconnect with your bigger sense of self, you will naturally engage in less self-comparison, and you won't feel as threatened by someone else's perceived wins or thrilled by their perceived losses. Your relationships will be strengthened, and you will be able to see the good in people beyond your perception of their looks. You will feel greater unity with other women and increased compassion for them and their personal choices and experiences in a culture of objectification.

The distraction and the lack of focus you feel doing absolutely anything, when part of your mental and physical energy is dedicated to monitoring and adjusting your body, clothes, makeup, and hair? That will diminish. You can regain your own dedicated attention and capacity to concentrate as you keep recognizing and rejecting that tendency to live in your head as you check off the boxes of your mental task list of self-objectification. You can experience a fully immersive flow state in which you are lost in a task or activity in a pure stream of focus. Anything you want to do well at or get better at will benefit from your undivided attention, free from unconscious body monitoring.

The pain that comes from rude comments, bullying, rejection in dating, and other hurts that might be connected to what others think of your looks? It will still hurt, but it won't crush you. When you can see more in yourself than just a body, appearance-related disruptions will not have the power to sink you or send you into punishing cycles of hiding and fixing. You can hold that pain in balance with the knowledge that you are in control of your self-perception and the understanding that other people's perceptions of you are shaped by objectifying ideals that you don't need to live up to. Others' views of you might even say more about how they feel about themselves. Their thoughts about you will not have the power over you that they used to. You will no longer blame yourself or try to control your body in order to control others' reactions to you. Beauty doesn't make you, so it can't break you, either.

All of the other body image disruptions—the sinking self-consciousness you feel when you catch your reflection or get tagged in a photo and you don't like what you see, or you don't fit into last year's pants, or your relative comments on your body, or you try on clothes in a fluorescently lit dressing room? They will sting, and that sting will cause you to turn against your body for a moment, splitting your identity in two: the one doing the looking and the one being looked at. But that sting and the splitting will be familiar reminders to come back to yourself, prompting you into action through practicing your skills for body image resilience. Rather than adapting to your body shame by turning back to your comfort zone, you can turn toward what you know about yourself and your capacity for growth and change. You will feel emboldened to leave your comfort zone because now you know to expect more out of your life and what you have to offer the world, regardless of how others might look at you.

In her book *Rising Strong,* resilience research superstar Brené Brown says, "Our job is not to deny the story, but to defy the ending—to rise strong, recognize our story, and rumble with the truth until we get to a place where we think, *Yes. This is what happened. This is my truth. And I will choose how this story ends.*"

You have the opportunity to choose a new ending to each and every one of your body image stories—every time you face a new disruption and choose how to respond. Rising with resilience and reuniting with your whole identity does not mean you are forever free from the pressures of an objectifying culture. It isn't possible to completely isolate yourself from the rest of the world, and if it were, it would be lonely and miserable.

It isn't realistic to think we can avoid the many reminders of the importance of beauty in our world. You probably still want to watch TV shows and movies as fun and mindless entertainment, even if they present women as parts to be admired. So do we. You will still spend time with friends, family, and colleagues—as you should—who aren't quite ready to question their participation in a culture of objectification. So do we. It is good and important to engage with the world and the people who aren't in the same place of understanding as you. You have opportunities to teach and model the liberation of being more than a body.

The goal shouldn't be to shun and judge everyone and everything that reflects objectifying ideas and images, but to instead make informed, critical, conscious choices about how you engage with such messages. The only way you can share your resources and your own examples of seeing more and being more is to stay connected and present in your culture and communities, even if—and especially if—harmful messages about bodies are reflected and reinforced there. Your goal should be to draw your own boundaries and recognize when objectification is seeping into your self-perception and pulling your body image out to sea.

Your Body Image Resilience Skill Set

As you have lived your life and faced difficulties and been changed (for better or worse) by them, you have been learning all along the way. You bring all of that experience and knowledge into your next body image disruption, and the next, and the next, and the next. That accumulation of understanding, skills, and sensitivities will buoy you up and power you forward as you find new ways to live and understand your body image and yourself. With those personal sources of wisdom and strength in tow, you can consciously and systematically practice your new skills for body image resilience in order to get you back home to yourself.

See more in your disruptions. As long as you are immersed in or in close proximity to a culture rife with objectification (which we all likely are), the waves of disruption to your body image won't stop. The pull to slip away from your grounded, whole self and dip back into the waters of objectification will probably never go away. Outside forces discriminate against you and work to oppress and objectify you — and they likely always will — but they don't have to divide you against yourself. Each body image disruption can sink you, subdue you, or spark something in you. When the wave hits, let the familiarity of that discomfort be your catalyst to immediately open your eyes and see more in that disruption. What is prompting your body shame right now? What are you feeling and thinking? Are you blaming your body for negative feelings or experiences that might not have anything to do with your body? Are you pinning your hopes and dreams and fears and anxieties on your body when the reality might be a bit more nuanced or complicated?

How are you tempted to cope with the shame and discomfort that might be stirred up through this disruption? It doesn't matter how many times you have consciously or unconsciously chosen the path of sinking deeper into shame or clinging to your uncomfortable comfort zone. Now that you can name your disruptions and your responses, you have the power and freedom to choose a new path guided by the knowledge that you are more than a body.

See more in your world. First, look at the messages about bodies that have created the body image conditions you're in now. What skills do you have to help you see more in your world? By now, you've begun to cultivate the ability to be discerning about every message you encounter about bodies, beauty, and worth—whether from mainstream media, social media, family, friends, church, school, or anywhere else. In the midst of a wave of shame, you can keep your head above water by first thinking carefully and critically about the sources that might be contributing to your ingrained ideas about your body. What ideals are you consciously or unconsciously holding yourself to? Who or what might benefit from you pinning your shame or hopes to your appearance? Looking through a lens of media literacy, what recent ideas, messages, or experiences may have skewed your body image perception?

How might you create a more habitable environment for your body image? It is likely that there are sources of beauty pressure (whether public or private, friend or stranger) that you can cut out, take a break from, or have a serious talk with. Consider what positive additions you can invite into your mental and physical space. What can you personally amplify, create, or contribute to remind yourself and others of your and their worth outside of their bodies?

See more in yourself. Look inside yourself. If self-comparison has taken a toll on your body image, you can drop your measuring stick and choose to self-reflect instead. Really get serious and honest with yourself about what you are thinking about yourself, why you are thinking it, and whether you can see things in another way. Turn toward people who can provide solidarity, advice, or professional help. Practice self-compassion to acknowledge and validate what you are experiencing. What would you tell your internal "little girl" in that moment? Mentally put your arm around that little you and reconnect to provide love and healing. Write down the thoughts you have for her, about who she is, what she is capable of, and what you want her to know about her body. If you've already written a message in the past, reread it. Meditate, walk, ponder, write, pray, practice yoga or tai chi, or whatever helps you personally tune into greater purpose and meaning in your life beyond your immediate physical self in order to reconnect with who you really are and what you are really capable of.

See more in each other. Next, extend your view outward to see more in others. If your self-comparison has warped your view of other people, you can choose to see them with compassion, recognizing your common humanity in this unfair, objectifying culture that puts pressure on us in so many ways. If your own or someone else's body commentary or dress-code policing has caused you pain, this is your chance to turn your compassion outward if necessary. In your interpersonal relationships, rethink the familiar reactions that might cause pain and instead try to err on the side of carefulness and love. You can move forward with others by extending kindness to all in your path, banding you together to have each other's backs as you navigate rough waters together.

See more in your health. When you start to feel that your whole value and identity rest on the way your body appears, you can take back your physical power by experiencing your body as an instrument, not an ornament. Watch out for misleading messages that conflate aesthetic ideals with fitness or health. If you follow those messages, your goals will depend on altering your weight, shape, size, and appearance, but often leave you far from your health and fitness hopes, sinking you into self-objectification and discouragement. Measure your health in terms of how you feel, what you can do, and what internal indicators tell you about how your body is doing. ***Use your body, regardless of how it appears, as an instrument for your own experience and benefit.***

See more in your self-help. Are you floundering in self-improvement that is rooted in self-objectification, focusing only on the visible parts of yourself? If advice and strategies to improve body image still point to a goal of "feeling beautiful," they might not be as transformative as you had hoped. Remember that self-help that relies on your objectification or how you are perceived by others isn't ultimately empowering or sustainable. Take control of your own empowerment by rooting out any beliefs and strategies that give you a false, temporary sense of self-worth and confidence by putting it in the hands of any other person, group, or industry. No one else can bestow your value or take it away. You have the power to be in control of your own sense of self, including your body image.

When each of these steps and skills is put into practice over and over again, every time you face a body image disruption, you can choose the life-changing path of rising with body image resilience that brings you home to yourself. Choosing this path changes you, causing you to grow and learn and move in ways that can be uncomfortable and even painful, but *never* as painful as hiding and fixing and sinking in the sea of objectification. Every disruption is an opportunity to opt out of self-objectification and to opt in to your body, your embodied wholeness.

The Privilege of Opting Out

Though we can't entirely opt out of the system that degrades us (because it will exist whether we want it to or not), we *can* opt out of the endless fight to find our worth and our confidence through that system. It is vital to recognize that any culture that views and values women as objects will continue to degrade and devalue us whether we are playing by its rules or not.

Buying into aspirational body ideals hasn't protected us yet. If we continue to buy into them and comply with those degrading rules about what women have to do to qualify to show up in this world, we will be complicit in guaranteeing that meaningful change *never* happens. If we resign to live as ornaments to be looked at because it is easier than fighting for a new way of being, we can be assured that our peers and younger generations will grow older with the same limited view of themselves and the same lifelong burden to carry by living to be looked at. The longer we continue to buy into and normalize the use of anti-aging solutions, lip injections, fillers, Botox, eyelash extensions, liposuction, breast augmentations, rhinoplasty, obsessive tracking of our calories/carbs/macros, and every other way we force our bodies and faces into compliance, we guarantee the next generation will do the same. What we do today is setting the bar of beauty expectations not only for ourselves, but also for those who look to us to see what it means to look normal and acceptable, let alone beautiful. This is a collective issue, which can be addressed only when we think beyond ourselves and our own choices and realize the kind of culture we are creating and reinforcing for generations to come.

It might be awkward. You might have to navigate some new territory in how you interact with other people as you make changes to your beauty routine and let go of restrictive diets and objectifying beliefs, but if you want to propel change in your own life or beyond, this is a task you must take on if you are able. Now is the time to recognize and exercise your power to be an example to others—loudly or quietly—of a woman who shows up and lives and loves regardless of whether she fits anyone else's ideals. The world needs women, and not just pretty visions of women hoping one day we'll qualify to be heard, to be seen, to lead. The world is desperate for you to show up now, not ten or fifty pounds from now. Your pain and shame—and the wisdom you've gained from becoming resilient through them—make you more of who the world needs you to be, not less.

You can choose to live as more than a body in lots of big and small ways. You can actively resist the pressure and temptation to "fix" your face and body, even when you might not fit the expressed or implied ideal. You can reject harmful beauty standards and the pressures to comply with them. You can show up. You can speak up. You can participate. You can lead. You can contribute and serve in all the ways you want and feel called to do. You can recognize and exercise your power to be present and live and love regardless of whether you fit anyone's expectations. You can prioritize your mental and physical wellness over your desire to fit arbitrary aesthetic ideals. So many others who are working to rise with body image resilience will support you. The revolution has begun.

If your relationship with your parents or other loved ones has been fraught with conflict because of comments about your body and their expectations for your appearance, talk to them. When they say something that makes you uncomfortable, tell them. Open up about the ways you are working on seeing yourself and other women as more than bodies, and tell them you want them to join you. Recommend things they can listen to and read to help reframe their thinking, which has likely been reinforced by their own parents and the entire culture in which they were raised. Give them the grace of realizing they have likely been steeped in objectification their whole lives, too, and it will take time to find their bearings in a world where women must be seen and treated as more than bodies. And while they are likely to express to you that they just want you to be happy, or find love, or keep your relationship, or avoid the body shame they have experienced, you can explain that you no longer want to be complicit in a world where only thin women's bodies are capable of love and respect and living free from shame. You are working to live your life free from those objectifying chains because you want to prove to yourself, to them, and to everyone else that happiness and love and success are possible in any body because we are more than bodies.

Look around: lots of people look lots of different ways and have lives filled with fulfillment, love, connection, success, health, and all the things you have learned to associate only with thinness, youthfulness, and narrowly defined sex appeal. Do not underestimate the power of looking around and seeing for yourself all the real-life examples who bust the myths about who deserves to be loved or happy. They are not hard to find. In your own life, can you think of people who don't fit all the beauty ideals or come anywhere close to them and are still successful, in loving relationships, respected, strong, confident, happy, healthy, or otherwise admirable to you? Could you be one of them? Are you willing to try?

If you can see the harms of objectification in your life, but you aren't willing to put in the work and make the hard choices and sacrifices to opt out of it for yourself, then meaningful change will not happen in your life, your family, your community, or your culture. If *you* don't fight against those forces and opt out of this rigged value system in all the ways you can, who will?

Must we wait and hope that our daughters (or future daughters) will figure this out? Should we just wait and cheer on our little sisters and nieces and cousins, our students, our friends, or the young women we lead and mentor while they watch us hide, lift, tighten, contour, liposuction, implant, diet, bleach, tan, laser, and otherwise fight against our natural, aging, growing, changing faces and bodies? If even the most privileged, confident, successful, forward-thinking, loved, and loving women are compelled to do those things, *why* wouldn't everyone else do the same?

What do you actually have to lose by opting out of our objectifying culture, even in small ways? Maybe taking a break from trying to reach those body ideals isn't the worst thing. Maybe weighing more than you do now or having different breasts than you did before you had children or showing your age or skipping the eyelash extensions or hair removal wouldn't *actually* decrease your quality of life. Especially if your income or employment won't be jeopardized by potential weight gain, a face that shows lines and expression, or hair that isn't expensively and time-consumingly colored, treated, and styled. Especially if you have a partner or a family or friends who love and support you.

For those who could *without a doubt* survive and maybe even thrive without all the buy-in to every beauty ideal, what do you have to lose? And what do you have to gain in its place? We want to propose that the things you fear about not living up to every beauty expectation are not as scary as you've been taught. Yes, some will face more repercussions than others. It might be hard. But being fat, or fatter than you are now, or older-looking than you look now, or having your natural hair color or texture, or being otherwise outside of the ideal is absolutely not the hellscape you have been led to believe. There is freedom and power on the other side.

We have personally proved this to be true in our own lives and will continue to cross our own boundaries that years of beauty norms have taught us are uncrossable. This is freedom. This is reimagining a whole new way of being by replacing the imaginary fantasy future version of ourselves with our actual, whole, embodied selves *right now.*

From Lindsay: I have proved every self-objectifying voice in my teenage and young adult mind wrong about what my body needed to look like in order for me to have a good life. At age thirty-three, after ten years of thinking that someday, when the circumstances were right, I might move to New York City, I faced the truth that the "right" circumstances in my mind included having a different body. Smaller. More worthy of living my ideal life and maximizing my potential there—in work, dating, making friends, and just walking down the street with confidence. Those distinct thoughts about needing to be thinner in my early twenties had evolved into deep, subconscious beliefs about what I deserved and what I qualified for. I was in a constant state of waiting until the circumstances were *right* without ever acknowledging that one of the things holding me back all these years was not thinking I *looked* right. When I imagined myself walking down the streets of Manhattan, I always envisioned a thinner self. That imaginary ideal put distance between the real me and who I thought I needed to be to thrive there, always pushing the reality of me moving there a bit further down the road. That imaginary ideal of my best NYC self went unchallenged until I proved to myself that it was nonsense—just another barrier holding me back while leaving me clinging to my uncomfortable, unchallenging, and unrewarding comfort zone.

During a few months of new and unexpected stress and dissatisfaction with my life in early 2019, I chose to put my belief in the power of resilience to work. I took my own skills and strategies for responding to body image disruptions and applied them to my general life disruptions. I began by dealing with my discomfort and discouragement directly rather than distracting or appeasing myself. I looked carefully at the environment I was surrounded by and what I had created for myself, including my full-time job, my longtime side gig with Lexie through our nonprofit, and my relationships. I assessed my beliefs about myself and others to see what faulty ideas were hurting my well-being, and I made some changes. I quit handling our nonprofit's social media to give myself some peace and time to disconnect. I started doing guided meditations and listening to affirmations every day in order to find balance and reconnect with myself. I started going to therapy and uncovered some previously unchallenged people-pleasing and perfectionist tendencies that were wreaking havoc on my well-being.

In April, my therapist asked me what I would do differently if I really lived my own life, putting myself first rather than prioritizing anyone else's feelings or perceptions of me. (This is admittedly easier to do when you are single and child-free, which I am.) I immediately said, "I've always wanted to move to New York," and surprised myself by bursting into tears and saying, "I don't even know why I'm crying about that." My therapist said, "I think you should consider doing that." I named some very practical hesitations. It only took two days for me to hit another anxious, frustrated low and start reflecting on ways to change my circumstances before I made the choice to move to NYC. As soon as the thought came into my mind, my stress dissipated and my decision was made.

I feel very fortunate that things fell into place smoothly, and six weeks later, I moved into my tiny Manhattan apartment and started a new full-time dream job. It has been one of the best decisions of my life, and I have experienced all of the transformational, eye-opening, exciting, stressful, romantic, challenging, and joyous moments while being as fat as I've ever been. I walk down the street every day looking much different from the Lindsay I imagined when I first dreamed of living in this city, and I am happy that I do. I proved my critical voice wrong. I challenged my worst fears and I won. *I am more than a body, and my life did not have to wait until my body caught up with my warped twenty-something ideals before I could be who I always wanted to be.*

Too many of us create arbitrary mile markers for ourselves that determine when we deserve some new experience or thing we've been wanting. *I'll go on that dreamy beach vacation once I can put on a swimsuit confidently. We'll get family pictures taken once I fit back into that outfit I would want to wear,* or, *when I don't look so much worse than my sister. I'll run for office or apply for that promotion or volunteer for that service project once I look like* this. Holding on to or even just unconsciously accepting these imaginary "goal" versions of ourselves is a way we create distance between ourselves and our bodies as well as our fullest lives. We think our "now" bodies are temporary impostors and our "future" bodies are who we *really* are, when we'll *really* be complete.

You can't heal the rift in your identity and reunite with your whole self if you are imagining a future self that isn't even real. Prove yourself wrong. Dash your long-held ideals about your body to pieces. Try to do the thing that makes you burst into tears when you acknowledge that you want to do it —regardless of how you look. Scale back on your beauty work and your attempts to change your body. See for yourself if you can survive it. Show others it is possible to take a break from the endless pursuit of a body ideal oasis and dry off. Give them permission to try. This is an act of resistance and a path to liberation, resilience, and a reunion, again and again, with your most complete self.

Keep in mind that not everyone is in the same position to opt out and push back on their own discrimination and objectification. What factors in your life might add to or detract from your privilege and the advantages you have in this world that elevates some people above others? Do you have a stable income and secure housing, a partner who loves you, an able body, freedom from racial or ethnic discrimination, or the ability to fit comfortably in an airplane or auditorium seat and easily find clothing that fits your body? Those of us who struggle with body image and the burden of objectification but still benefit from other forms of privilege need to humble ourselves, recognize our own advantages in a culture that values some bodies and faces above others, and make amends when we've perpetuated harmful ideals and hurtful messages.

Not all people can afford to reject beauty expectations or disengage from objectifying situations and people. If an employer has a bias against natural hair texture or styles and opting out of that unfair beauty standard might lead to losing her job, a woman might not be in a position to make a stand at that moment. If calling out harassment or rejecting a beauty standard or sexist uniform or expectation jeopardizes her safety, income, or opportunities, a woman is not in a position to demand change. If leaving a relationship with a partner who objectifies her would leave her homeless or with few resources, put her in a tenuous child custody situation, or potentially turn violent, a woman might not have the ability to get out of that demeaning relationship without help. Those of us who can take a stand owe it to our sisters who can't to try, even if it's uncomfortable or we face repercussions.

If you are in a relationship with someone who insists upon you meeting and upholding certain physical ideals, it is up to you to weigh the pros and cons of being with that person. Share your burden and ask for help carrying it. Tell them what you've learned about the harms of objectification and how it has impacted the way you feel about your body and yourself. Let them know that they are hurting you by doing things or saying things that feel objectifying. You don't deserve to be dehumanized in that way. Ask for compassion and understanding, and if they refuse, evaluate whether the relationship is actually in your best interest. Ask them to refrain from commenting on your appearance or others'—for the sake of yourself and those within earshot. Ask them to consider the impact of their own media choices, which might not only reflect harmful sexualized ideals of women in general but also perpetuate them in your home and daily life. Inform them about the negative impact their harmful comments and actions have on your life. When necessary, this could lead to distance from people who aren't supportive of your pursuit back to your whole self or who don't want to understand your perspective. Healthy romantic relationships are founded on love, respect, and attraction that extends far beyond the physical, and being in a relationship with a partner who values you as more than a body is crucial to your well-being. You do not deserve to be in a relationship with anyone who attempts to diminish you and divide you against yourself. You are whole. Surround yourself with people who encourage you to remain that way.

The reality is, we will all face repercussions from being objectified whether or not we choose to participate and buy into those ideals. Opting out of the endless fight to gain our worth through our beauty will not protect us from all the harms of our objectifying culture, but it can protect us from the toll that self-objectification takes on our lives and allow us to be our fully realized selves. It is a struggle worth having.

Having advantages that give you more freedom to push back on harmful ideas about bodies and beauty doesn't make it easy, but it does make it *easier*. We want to be very clear that those advantages do not inoculate anyone from body image issues or any of the pain and shame that come from objectification. In fact, in our experience, it is often the women who are closest to the cultural body ideals who experience some of the most predictable body image concerns. It seems like such a paradox that the most stereotypically beautiful women sometimes feel the most preoccupied with their "flaws." But when beautiful girls and women are praised, rewarded, and valued for their beauty—whether explicitly or implicitly—they learn that is what makes them valuable and powerful, and that they have to keep it up in order to hold on to their value. Beauty or thinness becomes a defining part of their identity and a source of some power. However, the unrealistic nature of those ideals and the very real nature of our aging, changing human bodies renders the currency of beauty of little value for any lasting period. It can be taken away as freely as it was given.

If you think you can't bear the thought of quitting your pursuit of an ideal body or opting out of some of the beauty work our culture asks women to do, ask yourself what you are really afraid of. Are you afraid of being rejected by your partner or future dating prospects? That's a possibility. But that is true regardless of how perfect you look. Beautiful actresses and models get dumped and cheated on all the time. Healthy relationships are founded on love, respect, and attraction that is much more than surface level. If your partner shames you or pressures you for not looking like you did when you met, they are dehumanizing you. Humans age and change and adapt, and we all need the freedom and acceptance to do that peacefully. Are you afraid of being mocked or criticized? You might be. But that is possible regardless of how you look. Celebrity beauty icons get trolled every day. The prettiest girls in school get bullied and harassed, too. Are you afraid of feeling like you have disappointed yourself or like you're letting yourself go? You might feel that way, but the truth is, you've only just found yourself. You are working on staying whole and grounded, and each time you slip outside of yourself as a distant observer, you can come back. You aren't a disappointment; you are a human doing the incredibly hard work of owning and embracing your full humanity.

It is important for each of us to get comfortable with letting ourselves down when it comes to our body ideals. Take some time to mourn the #bodygoals and objectifying hopes you're leaving behind and the nowhere destinations you spent so much time seeking. Process whatever emotions you need to process as you leave behind months or years or a lifetime of living to be looked at, or of waiting to live until you feel happy to be looked at. Let yourself really explore what you have lost and missed out on and the experiences and relationships that have been tarnished by objectifying ideals that you have internalized. What would you have done as a kid, a teenager, a young adult, or in any phase of life if you hadn't been hindered by unmet ideals, or burdened by maintaining the ideals you already met while carefully monitoring how others viewed you?

Igniting Your Fire

Learning about the objectifying, demeaning nature of the culture and beliefs you've grown up with can leave you feeling disillusioned. Realizing that self-objectifying thoughts and behaviors have held you back from fully living your life can be devastating. Letting go of your hopes for reaching an elusive "beauty ideal" destination can be strangely disappointing. And it can be hard to maintain relationships with people who are still chasing those ideals. *But pain and discomfort are actually required to access body image resilience because our "comfort zones" do not demand our improvement and growth.* Like poet and activist Gloria Anzaldúa so movingly put it, "'Knowing' is painful because after it happens I can't stay in the same place and be comfortable. I am no longer the same person I was before."

Seeing more in what you've always believed about your world and yourself can be a wave of disruption in itself. The first feeling you experience in your own path to rising with body image resilience might be annoyance — and it might even be directed at what we've written in this book. One woman wrote to us, saying:

> When I first started following your work, I caught myself being annoyed with some of your posts. And then, I finally realized why it bugged me. The problem was, you were discrediting everything I had been working so hard to accomplish. Decades of crash dieting, not-so-occasional tanning, image-driven exercise, hair extensions, Brazilian bikini waxes, Invisalign (for already pretty straight teeth), an extensive and expensive wardrobe, eyelash extensions, skin care products to make me look "younger" (at 23!), the list goes on and on. This all culminated in a consultation for a breast augmentation, therapy for an eating disorder, and a deviated septum surgery with some secretive shaping

of the nose. All this work, and you are telling me it doesn't matter? The thing is, I felt pretty. I like being pretty. And here you are, telling me that doesn't count for anything? It felt like a put-down. But you are doing me a favor. You are saying you don't care that I'm pretty. You are prying my worthless gold star from my desperate grip. It's like you've opened the door to the cell in which I've been bound and I'm cowering in the corner. One day I realized I had all the tools I needed to escape — I just had to stand up and walk out that door. I had to be willing, to be brave enough, to believe everything else I was — everything else I AM — is enough. So I did. I walked. And I've found that I'm actually pretty good at other things, which is much more fun than being pretty. I run without worrying about my love handles showing, an unflattering photograph doesn't ruin my day, and I get my hair wet. I always get my hair wet. Thank you for what you are doing. I didn't even know I needed you.

No matter what you're feeling when processing the ways objectification has impacted your life, know that it is okay. You might feel annoyance, or you might feel anger, sadness, or regret. Whatever it is, name it. Sit with it. It's okay to burn with rage or melt in sorrow that the value system you've bought into and sought after isn't the sure path to love and fulfillment you'd hoped for. Mourn the wasted time, energy, and money, the damaged relationships (with yourself and others), and unfulfilled goals and hopes that weight loss and beauty fixes couldn't deliver and prevented you from pursuing.

When you see the heavy costs and the toll this culture takes on you and your loved ones physically, mentally, and spiritually, deep, painful emotions are understandable and expected. You might know that your body is an instrument, while the outside world—even people and institutions you love and rely on—continues to see you as an ornament. Being objectified should be infuriating, and your fury will protect you from accepting and internalizing it. Your anger might not feel comfortable, and it might feel really out of place for the many women who have learned to suppress those feelings in favor of more subdued, pleasant, and self-sacrificing options. But rage and sadness aren't a bad or wrong way to feel about a cultural system that has inflicted real damage on so many of us, putting us at odds with our own bodies and sinking us into shame. Let those painful emotions fuel your fire to make progress and push for change—in your own life and for others.

Ask around and you'll find out that you aren't the only one who is pained and angry. The collective anger of women who are sick of submitting to dangerous ideals and watching themselves and others be reduced to objects is what we need to make real change. Don't excuse it or minimize it. Grapple with these feelings rather than dismissing them as negative or unproductive. Anger, sadness, and regret might be the signal that you are undergoing a revolutionary, enabling disruption that is propelling you toward a new, more fulfilling way of living. The objectification you experience in your life can motivate you and remind you to be more of who you are and who you could be. Not doubled, disembodied, and divided, but whole, embodied, and complete.

To stay reunited with yourself, you need to be united with other people for support. Calling out and eradicating objectification requires us to care about the collective and not just ourselves. No amount of validation, cultural approval, attention, online engagement, or personal good feelings is worth the collective disadvantage you perpetuate by uncritically accepting the objectifying conditions you're surrounded by. Every time we share something on social media about the harms of posting and viewing before-and-after weight-loss photos or complimenting people on their weight loss without knowing how or why it happened (among other topics that point out how objectifying ideals hold us back from actual health and happiness), we are hit with a barrage of people telling us to stop being jealous of women's progress and to just let people celebrate their "wins." We want people to understand that the harms of valuing and devaluing people based on their bodies still exist whether you personally feel the negative consequences or not. If we don't want beauty and body judgment to break us down, then we can't let it build us up either.

What we want people to understand is that when you accept or perpetuate objectifying ideals—because you personally benefit from the validation or you don't see the harm—you are simultaneously the oppressor and the oppressed. You are upholding an objectifying system that divides you against yourself as you slip outside of your body to evaluate it, and it also pushes everyone in your influence to divide against themselves, as you invite people to measure their value or their health by their appearance too. That same system keeps women at a disadvantage because we are judged and valued for our appearance more than men are, and held to even narrower ideals of thinness, youthfulness, and flaw-lessness that will always be just out of reach or at risk of slipping away. When you publicly or privately applaud people's bodies for getting closer to aspirational ideals, you keep yourself and other people content with their divided, disempowered reality as long as they feel the fleeting reward of external validation, or discour-aged and ashamed if they don't.

Trying to live and thrive in a world that so consistently reminds us that women are most valuable for their bodies is wildly diffi-cult. Can you imagine the impact of half the world's population feeling defined by and perpetually focused on their appearance as their primary source of value, health, happiness, and power? What is the world missing because a portion of our attention, effort, and income is devoted so consistently to our looks? How many girls and women in this world are being held back, wait-ing to really live until they feel qualified to be seen? How many are battling eating disorders, depression, and anxiety, undergoing painful procedures and complications while healing, and engag-ing in self-harm and self-loathing because of shame about their bodies? The impact is inconceivable. The lost presence and lead-ership and voice of women; the lost experiences of unencum-bered joy and fulfillment; the lost happiness, health, well-being, confidence; the damaged relationships and missed connections. What have you lost? What has your family, your community, your country, and the whole world lost? Alternatively, what does our whole world have to gain as more and more of us leave behind the paths that have asked us to shrink instead of grow?

More Than a Body Beach

As you reunite with yourself again and again, practicing coming back every time you slip by seeing more and being more, you not only heal your own body image and expand your possibilities, but you also help heal your community and expand its possibilities. Once you have found your footing and found yourself, you become another welcoming figure on the beach waving your sisters in. As you see others struggling to keep their heads above water in the sea, you call out to them, yelling words of encouragement to catch the next wave and head toward the beach. You might even cautiously venture out to meet one where she is, helping her more critically engage with the environment that surrounds you both and showing her a different way to understand her possibilities and herself. As she makes her way back, pushed by her own waves of disruption, you are excited to support her and bond over new ways of valuing and validating each other. You watch with joy as she is embraced by her higher self, the little girl she left on the beach all grown up.

Your community on the beach will grow as more voices and hands join yours in calling out and reaching out to those who are ready to grow instead of shrink and slip away. Envision waves of women reaching the shore, coming home to themselves, standing in their embodied, resilient power together. Our body image is an inseparable part of us that makes us stronger and more whole, not distressed and divided. The painful experiences and feelings you had at sea as you searched for fulfillment and belonging have made you more capable of discerning the difference between faux empowerment that hinges on others' reactions to your body and unwavering personal strength that grows from inside you. As you show up, engage, speak, create, innovate, move, lead, serve, love, and exist outside the confines of your fears of being looked at, you are reclaiming your power and your very existence. Together, we are creating a new, more habitable and joyful environment for ourselves and everyone else — one where we have the freedom and security that come from not just believing that our bodies look good, but knowing that our bodies *are* good, regardless of how they look. See you on the beach.

Final Questions

- How do you feel about your body?
- What truths have you learned or remembered about yourself throughout this book?
- What do you want to carry forward as you face disruptions that you can and can't anticipate right now?
- What do you know about your body and yourself that can help you choose the path to resilience again and again?

Acknowledgments

From Lindsay

Since this book represents so much more than the months it took to write, we owe many thanks to those who lent their support to our work over the years. Thanks to our mom, who lovingly and enthusiastically cheered from the sidelines at dozens of speaking engagements and still won't listen to our advice to avoid the comments sections of any story about us.

Thanks to my many friends who have provided not only encouragement and kindness, but especially distraction and entertainment while I disconnect from the sometimes overwhelming world of other people's body image burdens—thanks especially to Jackie, Ashley, Molly, Carly, Elizabeth, and to Jolyn, who passed away before I got to share this book in person. Thanks to the loyal crew of women who have followed our work since we first shared it on a crappy blog in 2009, and for those who have shared their body image transformations with us and shared our work with others.

Thanks to our agent, Terra, for finding us on her own search for mother-daughter body image advice, encouraging us to write a book, and walking us through the long process of bringing it to life. Thank you to our editor, Stephanie, and Houghton Mifflin Harcourt for investing in us as first-time authors.

And thanks to Lexie, who let me stay in her spare bedroom after I left NYC for the first three months of the COVID-19 pandemic, and only sent a couple of aggressive emails from the other room about making sure our workload was 50/50 while we made final revisions to this book. Mostly thank you to Lexie for giving me my two best little girl friends, Logan and Lane, and marrying an unbelievably supportive man who once secretly created a fake username to defend us in one of the comment sections our mom refused to ignore.

From Lexie

I'll start where Linds left off by acknowledging Trav, the man who is, as mentioned earlier, an unbelievably supportive husband and the best person I've ever known. Thank you for supporting me from the first time you saw me speak at an event before we'd even been set up on a blind date. Thank you for taking our babies away for weekends while I wrote and for being the kind of partner I never ever thought I'd be lucky enough to have.

And to my babies, Logan and Lane, I hope this book and all our work teaches you and reminds you that you are more. More than a body, more than cute, more than any descriptor for good or bad, more than you even know. I have all the hope that you and your generation will grow up striving to be more, not less.

To Linds, I'm so glad we could harness our powers for good

instead of the fiery competition to which we are so accustomed. Our work has brought us together, even when I had to email you a few times from the other room to make sure you were pulling your weight when our book deadline was approaching.

Because no parent can write a book or do much work at all without childcare, I must thank the village that helps us take care of our babies. To Ashley, Stephanie, Whitney, and Annalyse, I'm so grateful you have loved my girls like your own. It means the world to me.

And in a very twin-like fashion, I'd like to echo every word from Linds. To our parents, friends, our agent, publishing team, and the loyal friends and fans who have supported our work over the years, thank you so much! Your support means everything as we all rise with resilience together.

Notes

1. Rising with Body Image Resilience

20 *have intentionally injured themselves:* Martin A. Monto, Nick McRee, and Frank S. Deryck, "Nonsuicidal Self-Injury Among a Representative Sample of US Adolescents, 2015," *American Journal of Public Health* 108 (August 2018): 1042–1048, https://doi.org/10.2105/AJPH.2018.304470.

self-harm among ten- to fourteen-year-old girls: Melissa C. Mercado, Kristin Holland, Ruth W. Leemis, Deborah M. Stone, and Jing Wang, "Trends in Emergency Department Visits for Nonfatal Self-Inflicted Injuries Among Youth Aged 10 to 24 Years in the United States, 2001–2015," *Journal of the American Medical Association* 318, no. 19 (2017): 1931–1933, https://doi.org/10.1001/jama.2017.13317.

27 *"grow stronger through the disruption":* Glenn E. Richardson and Phillip J. Waite, "Mental Health Promotion Through Resilience and Resiliency Education," *International Journal of Emergency Mental Health* 4, no. 1 (2002): 65–75.

28 *The resiliency model:* Glenn E. Richardson, Brad L. Neiger, Susan Jensen, and Karol L. Kumpfer, "The Resiliency Model," *American Journal of Health Education* 21, no. 6 (1990): 33–39.

2. Critiquing and Creating Your Media Environment

43 *Geena Davis Institute on Gender in Media:* Geena Davis Institute on Gender in Media, "The See Jane 100: Gender and Race Representations in the Top Family Films of 2017," https://seejane.org/wp-content/uploads/see-jane -100-report-2017.pdf.

2016 report: Geena Davis Institute on Gender in Media, "The See Jane

Top 50: Gender Bias in Family Films of 2016," September 2016, https://seejane.org/wp-content/uploads/see-jane-top-50-gender-bias-in-family-films-of-2016.pdf.

44   *New York Film Academy:* Frank Pasquine, "Gender Inequality in Film," *New York Film Academy Blog,* November 2013, http://www.nyfa.edu/film-school-blog/gender-inequality-in-film.

In the highest-grossing films of 2018: Martha M. Lauzen, "It's a Man's (Celluloid) World: Portrayals of Female Characters in the Top Grossing Films of 2018," Center for the Study of Women in Television and Film, San Diego State University, February 19, 2019.

45   *Scholar Gaye Tuchman:* Gaye Tuchman, "The Symbolic Annihilation of Women by the Mass Media," in *Culture and Politics,* ed. Lane Crothers and Charles Lockhart (New York: Palgrave Macmillan, 2000): 150–174, https://doi.org/10.1007/978-1-349-62397-6_9.

50   *"the dissatisfaction industrial complex":* Tim Appelo, *"Dietland:* A Feminist Comedy That Hurts," *TV for Grownups,* AARP, June 1, 2018.

57   *Blue Chip Marketing Worldwide, described its success:* "Recharging Redness Relievers in a Beautiful Way," Effie, http://www.effie.org/case_database/case/SME_2019_E-462-326.

59   *chemical peels:* The Aesthetic Society, "Aesthetic Plastic Surgery National Databank Statistics 2019," https://www.surgery.org/sites/default/files/Aesthetic-Society_Stats2019Book_FINAL.pdf.

74   *Huge and powerful industries:* Diane E. Levin and Jean Kilbourne, *So Sexy So Soon: The New Sexualized Childhood and What Parents Can Do to Protect Their Kids* (New York: Ballantine Books, 2009).

79   *females in lead roles:* Geena Davis Institute on Gender in Media, "See Jane 2020 Film," https://seejane.org/wp-content/uploads/2020-film-historic-gender-parity-in-family-films-report-4.20.pdf.

99   *Natalie Muth:* Amanda Mull, "Putting Kids on Diets Won't Solve Anything," *The Atlantic,* August 20, 2019.

3. From Self-Objectification to Self-Actualization

103   *"She also exists outside":* Simone de Beauvoir, *The Second Sex* (New York: Vintage Books, 1989).

"self-objectification" in the late '90s: Barbara L. Fredrickson and Tomi-Ann Roberts, "Objectification Theory: Toward Understanding Women's Lived Experiences and Mental Health Risks," *Psychology of Women Quarterly* 21,

no. 2 (June 1997): 173–206, https://doi.org/10.1111/j.1471-6402.1997
.tb00108.x.

104 *regardless of age and background:* Rachel Calogero, "Objectification Theory,
Self-Objectification, and Body Image," in *Encyclopedia of Body Image and Human Appearance* Vol. 2, ed. Thomas F. Cash (San Diego: Academic Press,
2012): 574–80.

105 *"impossible to reach or maintain a flow state":* Fredrickson and Roberts, "Objectification Theory."
girls' activities and thoughts are more frequently disrupted: Barrie Thorne, *Gender
Play: Girls and Boys in School* (New Brunswick, NJ: Rutgers University Press,
1993).

106 *generally starts around puberty:* Elizabeth K. Hughes, Lisa K. Mundy, Hel-
ena Romaniuk, et al., "Body Image Dissatisfaction and the Adrenarchal
Transition," *Journal of Adolescent Health* 63, no. 5 (November 2018): 621–62,
https://doi.org/10.1016/j.jadohealth.2018.05.025.
it can start even younger: Steph Montgomery, "9 Ways Our Daughters Are
Objectified Before They Turn 5," *Romper*, November 15, 2017, https://
www.romper.com/p/9-ways-our-daughters-are-objectified-before-they
-turn-5-4246388.

113 *John Berger's 1972 book:* John Berger, *Ways of Seeing* (New York: Penguin
Books, 1972).

117 *American Academy of Facial Plastic and Reconstructive Surgery:* "American Academy of Facial Plastic and Reconstructive Surgery 2018 Annual Survey,"
American Academy of Facial Plastic and Reconstructive Surgery, January
23, 2019.

120 *one study showed:* The Renfrew Center Foundation, "Afraid to Be Your
Selfie? Survey Reveals Most People Photoshop Their Images," February 2014, https://renfrewcenter.com/news/afraid-be-your-selfie-survey
-reveals-most-people-photoshop-their-images.

122 *social comparison research about girls and women up to now:* Google Scholar
search terms, https://scholar.google.com/scholar?q=social+comparison+
among+women+and+girls&hl=en&as_sdt=0&as_vis=1&oi=scholart.
A whole body of research over decades: Gayle Bessenoff, "Can the Media Affect
Us? Social Comparison, Self-Discrepancy, and the Thin Ideal," *Psychology of Women Quarterly* 30, no. 3 (September 2006): 239–251, https://doi
.org/10.1111/j.1471-6402.2006.00292.x; Renee Engeln-Maddox, "Cognitive Responses to Idealized Media Images of Women," *Journal of Social
and Clinical Psychology* 24, no. 8 (December 2005): 1114–1138, https://doi

.org/10.1521/jscp.2005.24.8.1114; Inbal Gurari, John J. Hetts, and Michael J. Strube, "Beauty in the 'I' of the Beholder: Effects of Idealized Media Portrayals on Implicit Self-Image," *Basic and Applied Social Psychology* 28, no. 3 (2006): 273–282, https://doi.org/10.1207/s15324834basp2803_6; Emma Halliwell and Martin Harvey, "Examination of a Sociocultural Model of Disordered Eating Among Male and Female Adolescents," *British Journal of Health Psychology* 11, no. 2 (May 2006): 235–48, https://doi.org/10.1348/135910705X39214.

123 *"upward social comparisons":* Stephen L. Franzoi, Kris Vasquez, Katherine Frost, et al., "Exploring Body Comparison Tendencies: Women Are Self-Critical Whereas Men Are Self-Hopeful," *Psychology of Women Quarterly* 36, no. 1 (March 2012): 99–109, https://doi.org/10.1177/0361684311427028.

woman-vs.-woman competition: Christopher J. Ferguson, Monica E. Munoz, Sandra Contreras, and Krishna Velasquez, "Mirror, Mirror on the Wall: Peer Competition, Television Influences, and Body Image Dissatisfaction," *Journal of Social and Clinical Psychology* 30, no. 5 (May 2011): 458–483, https://doi.org/10.1521/jscp.2011.30.5.458.

126 *your self-consciousness is magnified:* Lyn Mikel Brown, *Raising Their Voices: The Politics of Girls' Anger* (Cambridge, MA: Harvard University Press, 1998).

127 *relationships between self-esteem and Instagram use:* Peta Stapleton, Gabriella Luiz, and Hannah Chatwin, "Generation Validation: The Role of Social Comparison in Use of Instagram Among Emerging Adults," *Cyberpsychology, Behavior, and Social Networking* 20, no. 3 (March 2017): 142–49, https://doi.org/10.1089/cyber.2016.0444.

133 *four steps of self-reflection:* Anthony M. Grant, John Franklin, and Peter Langford, "The Self-Reflection and Insight Scale: A New Measure of Private Self-Consciousness," *Social Behavior and Personality: An International Journal* 30, no. 8 (December 2002): 821–35, https://doi.org/10.2224/sbp.2002.30.8.821; M. F. Crane, B. J. Searle, M. Kangas, and Y. Nwiran, "How Resilience Is Strengthened by Exposure to Stressors: The Systematic Self-Reflection Model of Resilience Strengthening," *Anxiety, Stress & Coping* 32, no. 1 (2019): 1–17, https://doi.org/10.1080/10615806.2018.1506640.

143 *"Self-compassion means being more willing to experience difficult feelings":* Kristin Neff, "Meditation: Be Kind to Yourself," *Lion's Roar*, March 4, 2019, http://www.lionsroar.com/meditation-be-kind-to-yourself.

Belleruth Naparstek: Belleruth Naparstek, Health Journeys, http://www.healthjourneys.com.

150 *superstar musician Lizzo:* Lizzo, "Self-Care Has to Be Rooted in Self-Preservation, Not Just Mimosas and Spa Days," *Think*, NBC, April 19, 2019,
https://www.nbcnews.com/think/opinion/self-care-has-be-rooted-self
-preservation-not-just-mimosas-ncna993661.

156 *Swimming Upstream:* Laura Choate, *Swimming Upstream: Parenting Girls for
Resilience in a Toxic Culture* (Oxford, UK: Oxford University Press, 2016).

4. From Divided to United as Women

166 *as early as age six:* Joyce F. Benenson, "The Development of Human Female
Competition: Allies and Adversaries," *Philosophical Transactions of the Royal
Society B* (December 2013), https://doi.org/10.1098/rstb.2013.0079.

this manifests in everyday life: Tracy Vaillancourt, "Do Human Females Use
Indirect Aggression as an Intrasexual Competition Strategy?" *Philosophical Transactions of the Royal Society B* (December 2013), https://doi.org/10
.1098/rstb.2013.0080.

167 *decreased the odds by 25 percent for boys:* Lindsey S. Leenaars, Andrew V. Dane,
and Zopito A. Marini, "Evolutionary Perspective on Indirect Victimization in Adolescence: The Role of Attractiveness, Dating and Sexual Behavior," *Aggressive Behavior* 34, no. 4 (Jul-Aug 2008): 404–15, https://doi
.org/10.1002/ab.20252.

they deemed more attractive: Maria Agthe, Matthias Spörrle, and Jon K. Maner,
"Does Being Attractive Always Help? Positive and Negative Effects of At-
tractiveness on Social Decision Making," *Personality and Social Psychology
Bulletin* 37 (2011): 1042–54, https://doi.org/10.1177/0146167211410355.

less accepting of an apology: April E. Phillips and Cassandra Hranek, "Is
Beauty a Gift or a Curse? The Influence of an Offender's Physical Attractiveness on Forgiveness," *Personal Relationships* 19 (2012): 420–30, https://
doi.org/10.1111/j.1475-6811.2011.01370.x.

girls are more likely to be bullied: Melissa Seldin and Christina Yanez, *Student
Reports of Bullying: Results from the 2017 School Crime Supplement to the National
Crime and Victimization Survey* (NCES 2019-054), U.S. Department of Education (Washington, DC: National Center for Education Statistics, July
2019), https://nces.ed.gov/pubs2019/2019054.pdf.

these numbers doubled for overweight high school students: JoAnn Stevelos, "Bullying,
Bullycide and Childhood Obesity," Obesity Action Coalition, http://www
.obesityaction.org/educational-resources/resource-articles-2/childhood
-obesity-resource-articles/bullying-bullycide-and-childhood-obesity.

168 *classic study performed in the 1950s:* Stephen A. Richardson, Norman Goodman, Albert H. Hastorf, and Sanford M. Dornbusch, "Cultural Uniformity in Reaction to Physical Disabilities," *American Sociological Review* 26, no. 2 (April 1961): 241–47, https:/doi.org/10.2307/2089861.

   the three most common sources of friction: Deborah Tannen, *You're Wearing That? Understanding Mothers and Daughters in Conversation* (New York: Ballantine Books, 2006).

170 *A 2016 study:* Marisol Perez, Ashley M. Kroon Van Diest, Haylie Smith, and Michael R. Sladek, "Body Dissatisfaction and Its Correlates in 5- to 7-Year-Old Girls: A Social Learning Experiment," *Journal of Clinical Child & Adolescent Psychology* 47, no. 5 (2018): 757–69, https://doi.org/10.1080/15374416.2016.1157758.

182 *In a piece written for the* New York Times*:* Sara Clemence, "The Gender Divide in Preschoolers' Closets," *New York Times,* August 28, 2018, https://www.nytimes.com/2018/08/28/well/family/the-gender-divide-in-preschoolers-closets.html.

198 *view and value ourselves as objects:* Lexie Kite and Lindsay Kite, "Searching for Scraps of Power, One Swimsuit Pic at a Time," *Beauty Redefined,* January 21, 2018, https://beautyredefined.org/searching-for-scaps-of-power-swimsuit-pics.

199 *body-baring and tight clothing:* Marika Tiggemann and Rachel Andrew, "Clothes Make a Difference: The Role of Self-Objectification," *Sex Roles* 66 (2012): 646–54, https://doi.org/10.1007/s11199-011-0085-3.

200 *sexual objects in need of covering:* Lexie Kite and Lindsay Kite, "Female Objectification: Who's Really to Blame," *Beauty Redefined,* October 16, 2015, https://beautyredefined.org/objectification-leggings-blame.

5. Reclaiming Health and Fitness for Yourself

211 *World Health Organization has acknowledged:* WHO Expert Consultation, "Appropriate Body-Mass Index for Asian Populations and Its Implications for Policy and Intervention Strategies," *Lancet* 363 (2004): 157–63, https://doi.org/10.1016/s0140-6736(03)15268-3.

212 *come to be known as the BMI:* Ancel Keys, Flaminio Fidanza, Martti J. Karvonen, Noboru Kimura, and Henry L. Taylor, "Indices of Relative Weight and Obesity," *Journal of Chronic Diseases* 25, no. 6 (1972): 329–43, https://doi.org/10.1016/0021-9681(72)90027-6.

CDC website now states: Centers for Disease Control and Prevention, "About Adult BMI," 2018, https://www.cdc.gov/healthyweight/assessing/bmi/adult_bmi/index.html.

"inexpensive and easy for clinicians and for the general public": Centers for Disease Control and Prevention, "About Adult BMI."

in 2007: Traci Mann, A. Janet Tomiyama, Erika Westling, Ann-Marie Lew, et al., "Medicare's Search for Effective Obesity Treatments: Diets Are Not the Answer," *American Psychologist* 62, no. 3 (April 2007): 220–33, https://doi.org/10.1037/0003-066X.62.3.220.

again in 2013: A. Janet Tomiyama, Britt Ahlstrom, and Traci Mann, "Long-term Effects of Dieting: Is Weight Loss Related to Health?" *Social and Personality Psychology Compass* 7, no. 12 (December 2013), https://doi.org/10.1111/spc3.12076.

213   *Mann wrote:* Traci Mann, "Why Do Dieters Regain Weight?: Calorie Deprivation Alters Body and Mind, Overwhelming Willpower," *Psychological Science Agenda* (May 2018), https://www.apa.org/science/about/psa/2018/05/calorie-deprivation.

214   *In a large study of fourteen- and fifteen-year-olds:* Neville H. Golden, Marcie Schneider, and Christine Wood, "Preventing Obesity and Eating Disorders in Adolescents," *Pediatrics* 138, no. 3 (2016), https://doi.org/10.1542/peds.2016-1649.

direct result of an eating disorder: National Association of Anorexia Nervosa and Associated Disorders, "Eating Disorder Statistics" (2020), https://anad.org/education-and-awareness/about-eating-disorders/eating-disorders-statistics.

The number of children: Yafu Zhao and William Encinosa, "Hospitalizations for Eating Disorders from 1999 to 2006 : Statistical Brief #70," Agency for Healthcare Research and Quality (April 2011), https://www.hcup-us.ahrq.gov/reports/statbriefs/sb70.pdf.

215   *"this poisonous relationship":* Jessica Knoll, "Smash the Wellness Industry," *New York Times,* June 8, 2019.

217   *"Fitspo may be thinspo in a sports bra":* Charlotte Hilton Anderson, "Is 'Fitspiration' Really Any Better Than 'Thinspiration'?" *The Great Fitness Experiment,* February 26, 2012, http://www.thegreatfitnessexperiment.com/2012/02/is-fitspiration-really-any-better-than-thinspiration.html.

220   *how objectifying images affected female viewers:* Elizabeth A. Daniels, "Sex Objects, Athletes, and Sexy Athletes: How Media Representations of Women

Athletes Can Impact Adolescent Girls and College Women," *Journal of Adolescent Research* 24, no. 4 (May 2009): 399–422, https://doi.org/10.1177/0743558409336748.

230   *One fitness study of both men and women:* Anna Timperio, David Crawford, Amanda Telford, and Jo Salmon, "Perceptions About the Local Neighborhood and Walking and Cycling Among Children," *Preventive Medicine* 38, no. 1 (January 2004): 39–47, https://doi.org/10.1016/j.ypmed.2003.09.026.

231   *exercise bulimia:* Carrie A. Decker, "Exercise Bulimia—What's Healthy When It Used to Be a Problem?" *Eating Disorder Hope*, April 10, 2015, https://www.eatingdisorderhope.com/information/orthorexia-excessive-exercise/exercise-bulimia-whats-healthy-when-it-used-to-be-a-problem.

237   *Glenn A. Gaesser:* Marshall Terrill, "Big Fat Lies About Obesity: ASU Professor Says Health Risks of Obesity Have Been Exaggerated," *ASU Now*, January 29, 2019, https://asunow.asu.edu/20190129-discoveries-big-fat-lies-about-obesity.

        "only way to solve the weight problem": Linda Bacon, *Health at Every Size: The Surprising Truth About Your Weight,* second edition (Dallas, TX: BenBella Books, 2010).

239   *multiple studies have found that:* Terrill, "Big Fat Lies About Obesity."

        groundbreaking 2007 study: Xuemei Sui, Michael J. LaMonte, James N. Laditka, et al., "Cardiorespiratory Fitness and Adiposity as Mortality Predictors in Older Adults," *Journal of the American Medical Association* 298, no. 21 (December 2007): 2507–2516, https://doi.org/ 10.1001/jama.298.21.2507.

        "the harmful effect of fat just disappears": Phil Daoust, "Is It Healthier to Be Slim but Unfit or Fat and Fit?" *The Guardian*, March 9, 2010, https://www.theguardian.com/lifeandstyle/2010/mar/09/fit-fat-unfit-thin.

        Focusing on fitness rather than fatness: Centers for Disease Control and Prevention, "Division of Nutrition, Physical Activity, and Obesity at a Glance," August 7, 2019, https://www.cdc.gov/chronicdisease/resources/publications/aag/dnpao.htm; Joseph A. Knight, "Physical Inactivity: Associated Diseases and Disorders," *Annals of Clinical & Laboratory Science* 42, no. 3 (2012): 320–37.

240   *health problems often disappear or greatly improve:* Mayo Clinic Staff, "Exercise and Chronic Disease: Get the Facts," *In-Depth*, Mayo Clinic, December 18, 2018, https://www.mayoclinic.org/healthy-lifestyle/fitness/in-depth/exercise-and-chronic-disease/art-20046049; N. A. King, M. Hopkins, P. Caudwell, R. J. Stubbs, and J. E. Blundell, "Beneficial Effects of Exercise:

Shifting the Focus from Body Weight to Other Markers of Health," *British Journal of Sports Medicine* 43, no. 12 (September 2009): 924–27.

long-term study: Eric M. Matheson, Dana E. King, and Charles J. Everett, "Healthy Lifestyle Habits and Mortality in Overweight and Obese Individuals," *Journal of the American Board of Family Medicine* 25, no. 1 (2012): 9–15, https://doi.org/10.3122/jabfm.2012.01.110164

241   *brief for the APA:* Mann, "Why Do Dieters Regain Weight?"

strategy was successful: Joseph P. Redden, Traci Mann, Zata Vickers, Elton Mykerezi, Marla Reicks, et al., "Serving First in Isolation Increases Vegetable Intake among Elementary Schoolchildren," *PLoS One* 10, no. 4 (April 2015), https://doi.org/10.1371/journal.pone.0121283.

242   *"Dieting is against your best interests":* Christy Harrison, *Anti-Diet: Reclaim Your Time, Money, Well-Being, and Happiness Through Intuitive Eating* (New York: Little, Brown Spark Group, 2019).

252   *"feeling too fat to exercise":* David V. B. James, Lynne H. Johnston, Diane Crone, et al., "Factors Associated with Physical Activity Referral Uptake and Participation," *Journal of Sports Sciences* 26, no. 2 (May 2008): 217–24, https://doi.org/10.1080/02640410701468863; Kylie Ball, David Crawford, and Neville Owen, "Obesity as a Barrier to Physical Activity," *Australian and New Zealand Journal of Public Health* 24, no. 3 (May 2008): 331–33, https://doi.org/10.1111/j.1467-842X.2000.tb01579.x.

A study based on data from the 2002 National Physical Activity and Weight Loss Survey: Judy Kruger, Chong-Do Lee, Barbara E. Ainsworth, and Caroline A. Macera, "Body Size Satisfaction and Physical Activity Levels Among Men and Women," *Obesity* 16, no. 8 (September 2012): 1976–79, https://doi.org/10.1038/oby.2008.311.

256   *"When you're in the act of wanting something badly enough":* Autumn Whitefield-Madrano, *Face Value: The Hidden Ways Beauty Shapes Women's Lives* (New York: Simon & Schuster, 2016).

258   *"I realize now where all my insecurities started":* Amanda Trusty, "Bringing Body Love into Dance Class: A New Way of Teaching," *Huffington Post*, August 29, 2014, https://www.huffpost.com/entry/bringing-body-love-into-d_b_5732888.

259   *placed greater emphasis on their appearance attributes:* Ivanka Prichard and Marika Tiggemann, "Objectification in Fitness Centers: Self-Objectification, Body Dissatisfaction, and Disordered Eating in Aerobic Instructors and Aerobic Participants," *Sex Roles* 53, no. 1–2 (July 2005): 19–28, https://doi.org/10.1007/s11199-005-4270-0.

6. A Resilient Reunion

264 *"It's much, much worse than we ever envisioned":* Frederick Attewill, "Pressure on Girls for Perfect Body 'Worse Than Ever,' Says Orbach," *Agence-France Presse,* November 2018; Susie Orbach, *Fat Is a Feminist Issue* (New York: Paddington Press, 1978).

267 *The company's sales jumped from $2.5 billion to $4 billion:* Jack Neff, "Ten Years in, Dove's 'Real Beauty' Seems to be Aging Well," *AdAge,* January 22, 2014.

274 *"gay male gaze":* Mitchell J. Wood, "The Gay Male Gaze: Body Image Disturbance and Gender Oppression Among Gay Men," *Journal of Gay & Lesbian Social Services* 17, no. 2 (2004): 43–62, https://doi.org/10.1300/J041v17n02_03.

280 *2016 in-depth analysis:* Diana M. Zuckerman, Caitlin E. Kennedy, and Mishka Terplan, "Breast Implants, Self-Esteem, Quality of Life, and the Risk of Suicide," *Women's Health Issues* 26, no. 4 (2016): 361–65, https://doi.org/10.1016/j.whi.2016.03.002.

281 *More than 300,000 women:* American Society of Plastic Surgeons, "2018 National Plastic Surgery Statistics" (2019), https://www.plasticsurgery.org/documents/News/Statistics/2018/plastic-surgery-statistics-report-2018.pdf.

   increase from 1997: "ASAPS 1997 Statistics on Cosmetic Surgery," American Society for Aesthetic Plastic Surgery (1998), http://www.surgery.org/sites/default/files/ASAPS1997Stats_0.pdf.

Index